The American Psychiatric Association Practice Guideline for the Prevention and Treatment of Delirium

SECOND EDITION

Guideline Writing Group

Catherine Crone, M.D. (Chair)
Laura J. Fochtmann, M.D., M.B.I. (Vice-Chair; Methodologist)
Iqbal Ahmed, M.D.
Michele C. Balas, Ph.D., R.N., C.C.R.N.
Robert Boland, M.D.
Javier I. Escobar, M.D., M.Sc.
Thomas Heinrich, M.D.
Maga Jackson-Triche, M.D., M.S.H.S.
James L. Levenson, M.D.
Melissa Mattison, M.D.
Joseph McCullen Truett, D.O.
Mark A. Oldham, M.D.
Andreea Seritan, M.D.

Systematic Review Group

Laura J. Fochtmann, M.D., M.B.I. (Methodologist)
Seung-Hee Hong

Committee on Practice Guidelines

Daniel J. Anzia, M.D. (Chair)
R. Scott Benson, M.D.
Oscar Bukstein, M.D.
Catherine Crone, M.D.
Jacqueline Posada, M.D.
Ilse Wiechers, M.D.
Muniza Majoka, M.D. (Corresponding Member)
Saundra Stock, M.D. (Corresponding Member)
Michael J. Vergare, M.D. (Corresponding Member)
Laura J. Fochtmann, M.D., M.B.I. (Consultant)

APA Assembly Liaisons

Patrick Aquino, M.D.
Marvin Koss, M.D.
Brian Zimnitsky, M.D.
Lisa Schock, M.D.
Harold Ginzburg, M.D.
Jason W. Hunziker, M.D.

APA and the Guideline Writing Group especially thank Laura J. Fochtmann, M.D., M.B.I., Seung-Hee Hong, and Jennifer Medicus for their outstanding work and effort in developing this guideline. APA also wishes to acknowledge the contributions of other APA staff, including Kristin Kroeger Ptakowski. APA also thanks the APA Committee on Practice Guidelines (Daniel J. Anzia, M.D., Chair), liaisons from the APA Assembly for their input and assistance, and APA Councils and others for providing feedback during the comment period.

Note. The authors have worked to ensure that all information in this book is accurate at the time of publication and consistent with general psychiatric and medical standards, and that information concerning drug dosages, schedules, and routes of administration is accurate at the time of publication and consistent with standards set by the U.S. Food and Drug Administration and the general medical community. As medical research and practice continue to advance, however, therapeutic standards may change. Moreover, specific situations may require a specific therapeutic response not included in this book. For these reasons and because human and mechanical errors sometimes occur, we recommend that readers follow the advice of physicians directly involved in their care or the care of a member of their family

Second Edition

Manufactured in the United States of America on acid-free paper

29 28 27 26 25 5 4 3 2 1

American Psychiatric Association
800 Maine Avenue SW, Suite 900
Washington, DC 20024-2812
www.appi.org

Library of Congress Cataloging-in-Publication Data

Names: American Psychiatric Association, author, issuing body.
Title: The American Psychiatric Association practice guideline for the prevention and treatment of delirium / American Psychiatric Association.
Other titles: Practice guideline for the prevention and treatment of delirium
Description: Second edition. | Washington, DC : American Psychiatric Association, 2025. | Includes bibliographical references.
Identifiers: LCCN 2025006260 (print) | LCCN 2025006261 (ebook) | ISBN 9780890428030 (paperback ; alk. paper) | ISBN 9780890428016 (ebook)
Subjects: MESH: Delirium--therapy | Delirium--prevention & control | Practice Guidelines as Topic | Practice Guideline
Classification: LCC RC520.7 (print) | LCC RC520.7 (ebook) | NLM WM 204 | DDC 616.8/4--dc23/eng/20250430
LC record available at https://lccn.loc.gov/2025006260
LC ebook record available at https://lccn.loc.gov/2025006261t

British Library Cataloguing in Publication Data
A CIP record is available from the British Library.

Contents

Acronyms/Abbreviations

AHRQ = Agency for Healthcare Research and Quality
APA = American Psychiatric Association
ASA = American Society of Anesthesiologists
4AT = 4 'A's Test
bCAM = Brief Confusion Assessment Method
CAM = Confusion Assessment Method
CAM-ICU = Confusion Assessment Method for the Intensive Care Unit
CGI = Clinical Global Impression
CMS = Centers for Medicare & Medicaid Services
COVID-19 = coronavirus SARS-CoV-2 disease 2019
CTD = Cognitive Test for Delirium
3D-CAM = 3-Minute Diagnostic Interview for the Confusion Assessment Method
DDT-Pro = Delirium Diagnostic Tool-Provisional
DOSS = Delirium Observation Screening Scale
DRS = Delirium Rating Scale
DRS-R-98 = Delirium Rating Scale—Revised-98
DSM-III-R = *Diagnostic and Statistical Manual of Mental Disorders*, 3rd Edition, Revised
DSM-IV = *Diagnostic and Statistical Manual of Mental Disorders*, 4th Edition
DSM-5 = *Diagnostic and Statistical Manual of Mental Disorders*, 5th Edition
DSM-5-TR = *Diagnostic and Statistical Manual of Mental Disorders*, 5th Edition, Text Revision
DTS = Delirium Triage Screen
ECG = electrocardiogram
ECT = electroconvulsive therapy
EEG = electroencephalogram
EHR = electronic health record
GAD-7 = Generalized Anxiety Disorder-7
GRADE = Grading of Recommendations Assessment, Development and Evaluation
GWG = Guideline Writing Group
HIE = health information exchange
ICDSC = Intensive Care Delirium Screening Checklist
ICU = intensive care unit
MDAS = Memorial Delirium Assessment Scale
MMSE = Mini-Mental State Examination
MoCA = Montreal Cognitive Assessment
NH-CAM = Nursing Home Confusion Assessment Method
NMS = neuroleptic malignant syndrome
NuDESC = Nursing Delirium Screening Scale
PHQ-9 = Patient Health Questionnaire-9
PMDP = prescription monitoring data program
PTSD = posttraumatic stress disorder
RASS = Richmond Agitation-Sedation Scale
RCT = randomized controlled trial
SLUMS = Saint Louis University Mental Status
SRG = Systematic Review Group
WHODAS 2.0 = World Health Organization Disability Assessment Schedule 2.0
WHOQOL-BREF = World Health Organization Quality of Life BREF

Introduction

Rationale

The goal of this guideline is to prevent the development of delirium in at-risk individuals and to improve the quality of care and treatment outcomes for patients with delirium.

The prevalence rates of delirium range widely depending on the patient population and treatment setting (e.g., age, hospital vs. outpatient setting, medical vs. cardiac unit, surgical vs. critical care unit). In emergency department settings, delirium is present in up to one-third of patients, depending on age and referral source, but is often unrecognized (F. Chen et al. 2022; Lee et al. 2022; Oliveira JE Silva et al. 2021; O'Regan et al. 2018). However, most data on the incidence and prevalence of delirium come from hospitalized patients and often older adults (typically age 65 and older) rather than from the community (Ospina et al. 2018). A meta-analysis of 33 studies of adults (age 18 and older) on medical inpatient units reported an overall delirium occurrence rate of 23% (Gibb et al. 2020). In older adults on medical inpatient units, 11%–25% will have delirium on admission, with an additional 29%–31% developing delirium during the hospital stay (Vasilevskis et al. 2012). The pooled prevalence of delirium among adults in intensive care units (ICUs) has been estimated at 31%, with a pooled incidence of 4%–11% depending on delirium motor subtype (Krewulak et al. 2018). In mechanically ventilated patients in ICUs, who are typically sedated and seriously ill, delirium appears to be extremely common, with an estimated prevalence of 75% (Mart et al. 2021). With postoperative patients, rates of delirium increase with the severity of the surgery (Vasilevskis et al. 2012). In patients undergoing cardiovascular surgery, the prevalence of postoperative delirium ranges from approximately 7% to 51%, depending on the type of surgery and the rating method used (Cai et al. 2022; Wilson et al. 2020). Delirium also occurs in ambulatory settings. For example, among older adult outpatients of a memory clinic in a psychiatric hospital (Quispel-Aggenbach et al. 2021), the rate of probable delirium was 19%. The prevalence of delirium in palliative care populations also varies widely, from a low of 4% to a high of 88%, based on care setting and stage of illness (Wilson et al. 2020).

Since 2020, increasing research has been exploring the neuropsychiatric side effects of infection with coronavirus SARS-CoV-2 disease 2019 (COVID-19), including manifestations of delirium. In hospitalized patients with COVID-19, delirium is common (Duggan et al. 2021; Wong et al. 2022) and may precede the onset of hypoxia, organ failure, acute respiratory failure, or other severe illnesses (Kotfis et al. 2020). A review of 48 observational studies of patients with COVID-19 found that delirium was present on hospital admission in 28% of individuals age 65 and older and in almost 16% of individuals younger than 65 (Peterson et al. 2021). Delirium incidence while hospitalized with COVID-19 was also common, with 25% of those age 65 and older and 71% of those younger than 65 experiencing delirium (Peterson et al. 2021). Among 77 case reports, case series, or observational cohorts, 65%–80% of COVID-19 patients admitted to the ICU had delirium (Hawkins et al. 2021). Similarly, 75% of critically ill cancer patients with COVID-19 had delirium (Bjerre Real et al. 2022). Particularly in the early stages of the pandemic, a myriad of social, epidemiological, iatrogenic, and psychological factors unique to COVID-19 were hypothesized to play a role in the development and exacerbation of delirium in COVID-19 patients (Kotfis et al. 2020). These included, but were not limited to, social isolation and loneliness related to quarantine procedures, anxiety and fear surrounding the effect of the global pandemic, staff shortages and high levels of stress in health care professionals, increased use of sedative and antipsychotic medication to reduce patient distress, prolonged mechanical ventilation with sedation and immobilization, and delayed extubation because of concerns about aerosol spread of the virus (Inouye 2021; Kotfis et al. 2020; Pun et al. 2021). However, it is unclear whether these findings and contributors to delirium from earlier in the COVID-19 pandemic will hold true in future cases of COVID-19 and other infectious diseases.

Delirium exacts a significant economic toll on individuals, their families, and society because of factors such as lengthy hospital stays, ICU admissions, rehospitalizations, and lost wages from work absenteeism (Gou et al. 2021; Kinchin et al. 2021; Vasilevskis et al. 2018). In the United States, direct health care costs of hospitalized older adults with delirium are significantly higher than those of hospitalized patients without delirium, even after adjusting for demographic and clinical covariates; however, significant heterogeneity exists in study designs, which complicates assessments of economic impact (Caplan et al. 2020; Kinchin et al. 2021). Estimates based on data from the late 1990s and reported in 2005 dollars suggested that the total 1-year attributable costs of delirium among older adults in the United States ranged from $143 billion to $152 billion per year nationally (Leslie et al. 2008). For hospitalized inpatients, added costs due to delirium have been estimated at $6.6 billion to $82.4 billion annually in the United States alone based on 2019 data (Kinchin et al. 2021). Direct 1-year health care costs of postoperative delirium specifically have been estimated at $32.9 billion per year based on data from 2019 (Gou et al. 2021). Patients with hyperactive delirium are estimated to need at least 240 minutes of additional personnel time expended each day of hospitalization (Weinrebe et al. 2016). Additionally, the 30-day incremental cumulative cost of delirium treated in the ICU is approximately $18,000, or an additional $600 per day (Vasilevskis et al. 2018). These costs are almost certainly an underestimate because of the significant mortality rates of patients with delirium in ICU settings (Vasilevskis et al. 2018).

Mortality and morbidity associated with delirium are both substantial in many patient populations. Delirium has been associated with increased mortality during general medical and critical care hospitalization (Hshieh et al. 2020) and more specifically with a 38% increase in the risk of death (Maldonado 2017). Postsurgical delirium has been reported to have a 30-day mortality rate of up to 10% compared with 1% in postsurgical patients without delirium (Jin et al. 2020). Delirium was a significant independent predictor of mortality at 30 days, 90 days, 6 months, and 12 months in a population of Medicare beneficiaries discharged from the emergency department (Israni et al. 2018). At 30 days, mortality among patients with delirium was nearly five times higher than in patients without delirium, even after adjusting for age, sex/gender, dementia[1] diagnosis, and Charlson Comorbidity Index score (Israni et al. 2018). Delirium also increases the risk of death among patients with COVID-19, with a pooled mortality risk (44%) that is triple that of COVID-19 patients without delirium (Peterson et al. 2021). Among ICU patients, it is less clear whether delirium has an independent effect on short- or long-term mortality (Andrews et al. 2020; Duprey et al. 2020; Fiest et al. 2021; Hughes et al. 2021; Klein Klouwenberg et al. 2014; Li et al. 2022, 2023; Rood et al. 2019; Salluh et al. 2015; Sanchez et al. 2020; Wolters et al. 2014). Instead, apparent differences in mortality may relate to factors such as delirium subtype (Hughes et al. 2021; Rood et al. 2019), days of delirium or coma (Andrews et al. 2020; Duprey et al. 2020; Li et al. 2022), presence of frailty (Sanchez et al. 2020), or the tool used to assess for the presence of delirium (Li et al. 2023).

Delirium has been linked to a host of deleterious outcomes and complications, including increased hospital and ICU lengths of stay, greater risk of rehospitalization, more time spent on mechanical ventilation, increased odds of cognitive dysfunction, greater frailty and risk of falls, persistent functional decline, greater likelihood of discharge to long-term-care facilities rather than to home, increased risk of respiratory and neurological sequelae, and higher odds of difficult

[1]Although DSM-5-TR uses the term *major neurocognitive disorder,* in this guideline, the term *dementia* is used for consistency with most clinical use and published literature.

and extended extubation (Fiest et al. 2021; Goldberg et al. 2020; Haley et al. 2019; Inouye et al. 2016; Kinchin et al. 2021; Maldonado 2017). Even after remission, patients can continue to experience protracted cognitive impairment, ongoing functional decline, a heightened mortality risk, subsequent rehospitalizations and emergency department visits, and an increased need for long-term care (Fiest et al. 2021; Goldberg et al. 2020; Inouye et al. 2016; Kukreja et al. 2015; Richardson et al. 2021; Salluh et al. 2015; Wolters et al. 2014).

Delirium may be a significant strain on patients and caregivers. Contributors include psychosocial distress, such as anxiety and fear, and the high costs and health care needs associated with co-occurring conditions (e.g., Alzheimer's dementia, other end-stage diseases) (Fong et al. 2019). Delirium-related distress in patients—which may include posttraumatic stress disorder (PTSD)–like symptoms, anxiety, and depression—appears associated with increased severity of the underlying critical illness, greater cognitive impairment, and longer duration of delirium (MacLullich et al. 2022; Williams et al. 2020). Furthermore, psychosocial consequences of distress during delirium, such as delirium recall or memories, may be upsetting to patients and may persist for months after the condition resolves (Williams et al. 2020). Family members also may report experiencing fear, anxiety, depression, and PTSD-like symptoms from observing their loved one's struggle with cognitive decline, emotional lability, motor disturbances, and disorientation (Rosgen et al. 2021; Williams et al. 2020).

For all these reasons, this practice guideline focuses on preventing the development of delirium in at-risk individuals and improving the quality of care for patients with delirium, thereby reducing the mortality, morbidity, and significant psychosocial and health consequences of this important psychiatric condition.

Scope of Document

This practice guideline focuses on evidence-based nonpharmacological and pharmacological interventions to prevent or treat delirium in adults. In addition, it includes statements related to assessment and treatment planning, which are an integral part of patient-centered care. The scope of this document is shaped by the diagnostic criteria for delirium, with a particular focus on delirium as defined by the *Diagnostic and Statistical Manual of Mental Disorders*, 5th Edition, Text Revision (DSM-5-TR; American Psychiatric Association 2022). Unless otherwise specified, when the term *delirium* is used in this practice guideline, it should be understood in a generic sense. Our comments pertain to delirium due to any cause with the exception of delirium related to withdrawal from alcohol or sedative, hypnotic, or anxiolytic medications, which represents a physiologically discrete condition. As such, alcohol withdrawal delirium and delirium due to withdrawal from sedative, hypnotic, or anxiolytic medications have their own clinical assessment and treatment implications, which are often different from the management of delirium due to other causes. Although other physiologically discrete conditions are likely to present with delirium, this practice guideline does not differentiate these conditions because the literature in support of physiological subtypes of delirium remains in its early stages (Bowman et al. 2024). Our comments are also limited by the available evidence, as obtained by a systematic review of the literature through July 9, 2021.

Although this guideline and the associated systematic review have been limited to adults, delirium does occur in children and adolescents. It is prevalent in pediatric critical care settings (Semple et al. 2022), and risk factors for delirium and potential interventions in children and adolescents differ from those for adults. Consequently, the reader is directed to guidelines and reviews on pediatric delirium for additional information on this important topic (Harris et al. 2016; Ista et al. 2023; Kim et al. 2024; Silver et al. 2019; H.A.B. Smith et al. 2022).

Most studies that were identified in the systematic review for this guideline included patients older than 50 and generally older than 65. Research participants were predominantly male, but in many studies, the sample was nearly evenly divided. However, studies of much older adults (age

85 and older) tended to have a predominance of female participants. Studies that specified gender divided the sample into males and females without reporting information on other genders. Most studies also enrolled predominantly White participants or did not specify the racial, ethnic, or cultural characteristics of the sample. Study populations were typically drawn from ICUs or other inpatient hospital settings (e.g., general medical unit, postsurgical unit, cardiac unit), although some studies focused specifically on populations in long-term-care facilities, such as nursing homes. These limitations of the evidence emphasize the compelling need for additional research in more representative samples, and these limitations should be considered in terms of the document scope. Studies also typically did not specify patients' baseline level of cognitive functioning, making it difficult to know whether findings are applicable to all individuals with delirium.

Although delirium may present as hypoactive, hyperactive, or with a mixed level of activity, studies typically did not describe whether patients had a motor subtype of delirium. Individuals with hypoactive delirium likely were identified less often and, thus, were less likely to be represented in the evidence base. Also, comatose patients may have been viewed as having hypoactive delirium, influencing the study findings (European Delirium Association and American Delirium Society 2014; Oldham et al. 2017). Medication-related sedation also may resemble delirium in some patients. Furthermore, in contrast to DSM-5 (American Psychiatric Association 2013), DSM-5-TR (American Psychiatric Association 2022) now notes that an inability to respond to verbal or physical stimulation should be classified as an arousal disorder such as coma or stupor, and not delirium. The degree of arousal and the motor subtype of delirium may also influence the effects of interventions; misclassification might therefore alter study conclusions.

It is important to note that the term *delirium* can overlap with related terms that represent clinically distinct entities and concepts. For example, *acute encephalopathy* describes generalized pathophysiology of the brain that develops rapidly (i.e., in less than 4 weeks) (Slooter et al. 2020). It can present as subsyndromal delirium or delirium (as well as coma) but may include additional features that are not part of the clinical picture of delirium, such as seizures and extrapyramidal signs (Slooter et al. 2020). As opposed to acute encephalopathy, which lacks a strict clinical definition, the term *delirium* is a clinical syndrome identified during clinical assessment of the patient. It has been recommended that terms including *acute confusional state, acute brain dysfunction, acute brain failure,* and *altered mental status* no longer be used (Slooter et al. 2020), especially when a more specific diagnosis can be given; these terms were also viewed as being outside the scope of this guideline.

Our systematic review did not include studies on delirium related to withdrawal from alcohol or sedative, hypnotic, or anxiolytic medications because this condition differs in etiology, assessment, and treatment from other types of delirium. Studies on risk factors for delirium were also outside the scope of our systematic review, although we conducted targeted searches on delirium risk factors, and this topic has been reviewed by others (Bramley et al. 2021; Ormseth et al. 2023; Zaal et al. 2015). We also did not examine the effect of potential moderators of interventions for delirium because these were not reported consistently or in relation to primary outcomes. These moderators, including social determinants of health and effects of health disparities (Arias et al. 2022; Boltz et al. 2021; Reppas-Rindlisbacher et al. 2022; Wu et al. 2021), are important areas for further study. Although treatment-related costs are often barriers to receiving treatment, costs of treatment typically differ by country and geographic region and vary widely within the health care system and payment model. Consequently, cost-effectiveness and reimbursement considerations are also outside the scope of this guideline.

Overview of the Development Process

Since the publication of the Institute of Medicine (now known as the National Academy of Medicine) report *Clinical Practice Guidelines We Can Trust* (Institute of Medicine 2011), there has been an increasing focus on using clearly defined, transparent processes for rating the quality of evidence and the strength of the overall body of evidence in systematic reviews of the scientific literature. This guideline was developed using a process intended to be consistent with the recommendations of the Institute of Medicine (2011) and the *Principles for the Development of Specialty Society Clinical Guidelines* of the Council of Medical Specialty Societies (2017). Parameters used for the guideline's systematic review are included with the full text of the guideline and in Appendix B; the general development process is described in the following document available at the American Psychiatric Association (APA) website: https://www.psychiatry.org/psychiatrists/practice/clinical-practice-guidelines/guideline-development-process.

APA is committed to mitigating the mental health inequities that prevent individuals from fully benefiting from preventive services and treatment. Systemic and structural racism results in policies and practices, including health care delivery, that can lead to inequities. APA recognizes that race, ethnicity, and gender are all social constructs, which are complex and multidimensional variables. These variables can inform social determinants of health, which are important for health risks and mental health outcomes. Throughout its work, the APA is committed to helping to reverse the negative effects of systemic and structural racism, gender-based discrimination, and other sources of bias in health inequities and their effects on mental health status and health care delivery.

Rating the Strengths of Guideline Statements and Supporting Research Evidence

Development of guideline statements entails weighing the potential benefits and harms of the statement and then identifying the level of confidence in that determination. This concept of balancing benefits and harms to determine guideline recommendations and strength of recommendations is a hallmark of GRADE (Grading of Recommendations Assessment, Development and Evaluation), which is used by multiple professional organizations around the world to develop practice guideline recommendations (Guyatt et al. 2013). With the GRADE approach, recommendations are rated by assessing the confidence that the benefits of the statement outweigh its harms and burdens, determining the confidence in estimates of effect as reflected by the quality of evidence, estimating patient values and preferences (including whether they are similar across the patient population), and identifying whether resource expenditures are worth the expected net benefit of following the recommendation (Andrews et al. 2013).

In weighing the balance of benefits and harms for each statement in this guideline, our level of confidence is informed by available evidence, which includes evidence from clinical trials as well as expert opinion and patient values and preferences. Evidence for the benefit of a particular intervention within a specific clinical context is identified through systematic review and is then balanced against the evidence for harms. In this regard, *harms* are broadly defined and may include serious adverse events, less serious adverse events that affect tolerability, minor adverse events, negative effects of the intervention on quality of life, barriers and inconveniences associated with treatment, direct and indirect costs of the intervention (including opportunity costs), and other negative aspects of the treatment that may influence decision-making by the patient, the clinician, or both.

Many topics covered in this guideline have relied on forms of evidence such as consensus opinions of experienced clinicians or indirect findings from observational studies rather than research from randomized trials. It is well recognized that there are guideline topics and clinical circumstances for which high-quality evidence from clinical trials is not possible or is unethical to obtain (Council of Medical Specialty Societies 2017). For example, many questions need to be asked as part of an assessment, and inquiring about a particular symptom or element of the history cannot be separated out for study as a discrete intervention. It would also be impossible to separate changes in outcomes due to assessment from changes in outcomes due to ensuing treatment. Research on psychiatric assessments and some psychiatric interventions can also be complicated by multiple confounding factors, such as the interaction between the clinician and the patient or the patient's unique circumstances and experiences. The GRADE working group and guidelines developed by other professional organizations have noted that a strong recommendation or "good practice statement" may be appropriate even in the absence of research evidence when sensible alternatives do not exist (Andrews et al. 2013; Brito et al. 2013; Djulbegovic et al. 2009; Hazlehurst et al. 2013). For each guideline statement, we have described the type and strength of the available evidence, as well as the factors, including patient preferences, that were used in determining the balance of benefits and harms.

The Guideline Writing Group (GWG) determined ratings of strength of the statement (i.e., recommendation or suggestion) by a modified Delphi method using blind, iterative voting and discussion. In order for the GWG members to be able to ask for clarifications about the evidence, the wording of statements, or the process, the vice-chair of the GWG served as a resource and did not vote on statements. The chair and other formally appointed GWG members were eligible to vote. In weighing potential benefits and harms, GWG members considered the strength of supporting research evidence, their own clinical experiences and opinions, and patient preferences. For recommendations, at least 11 of 12 members must have voted to recommend the intervention or assessment after three rounds of voting, and at most 1 member was allowed to vote other than to "recommend" the intervention or assessment. On the basis of the discussion among the GWG members, adjustments to the wording of guideline statements could be made between the voting rounds. If this level of consensus was not achieved, the GWG could have agreed to make a suggestion rather than a recommendation. No suggestion or statement could have been made if 3 or more members voted "no statement." Differences of opinion within the GWG about ratings of strength of recommendation, if any, are described for each statement in Appendix F.

A *recommendation* (denoted by the numeral 1 after the guideline statement) indicates confidence that the benefits of the intervention clearly outweigh the harms (see Table 1). A *suggestion* (denoted by the numeral 2 after the guideline statement) indicates greater uncertainty. Although the benefits of the statement are still viewed as outweighing the harms, the balance of benefits and harms is more difficult to judge, or either the benefits or the harms may be less clear. With a suggestion, patient values and preferences may be more variable, and this can influence the clinical decision that is ultimately made. When a negative statement is made, ratings of strength of recommendation should be understood as meaning the inverse of the above (i.e., *recommendation* indicates confidence that harms clearly outweigh benefits). In addition, these strengths of recommendation correspond to ratings of *strong* or *weak* (also termed *conditional*), as defined under the GRADE method for rating recommendations in clinical practice guidelines (described in publications such as Guyatt et al. 2008 available on the GRADE Working Group website at: www.gradeworkinggroup.org).

Each guideline statement also has an associated rating for the *strength of supporting research evidence*. Three ratings are used—*high*, *moderate*, and *low* (denoted by the letters A, B, and C, respectively)—and reflect the level of confidence that the evidence for a guideline statement reflects a true effect based on consistency of findings across studies, directness of the effect on a specific health outcome, precision of the estimate of effect, and risk of bias in available studies (Agency for Healthcare Research and Quality 2014; Balshem et al. 2011; Guyatt et al. 2006). These ratings were determined by the methodologist (L.J.F.) and reviewed by members of the Systematic Review Group and GWG.

Disclaimer

The APA Practice Guidelines are assessments of current (as of the date of authorship) scientific and clinical information provided as an educational service. The guidelines 1) do not set a standard

Table 1 Rating the strengths of guideline statements and evidence for guideline statements

Strength of guideline statement			Strength of evidence		
1	Recommendation	Denotes confidence that the benefits of the intervention clearly outweigh the harms.	A	High confidence	Further research is very unlikely to change the estimate of effect and our confidence in it.
2	Suggestion	Denotes benefits that are viewed as outweighing harms, but the balance is more difficult to judge, and patient values and preferences may be more variable.	B	Moderate confidence	Further research may change the estimate of effect and our confidence in it.
			C	Low confidence	Further research is likely to change the estimate of effect and our confidence in it.

of care and are not inclusive of all proper treatments or methods of care; 2) are not continually updated and may not reflect the most recent evidence, because new evidence may emerge between the time information is developed and when the guidelines are published or read; 3) address only the question(s) or issue(s) specifically identified; 4) do not mandate any particular course of medical care; 5) are not intended to substitute for the independent professional judgment of the treating clinician; and 6) do not account for individual variation among patients. As such, it is not possible to draw conclusions about the effects of omitting a particular recommendation, either in general or for a specific patient. Furthermore, adherence to these guidelines will not ensure a successful outcome for every individual, nor should these guidelines be interpreted as including all proper methods of evaluation and care or excluding other acceptable methods of evaluation and care aimed at the same results. The ultimate recommendation regarding a particular assessment, clinical procedure, or treatment plan must be made by the clinician directly involved in the patient's care in light of the psychiatric evaluation, other clinical data, and the diagnostic and treatment options available. Such recommendations should be made in collaboration with the patient whenever possible and should incorporate the patient's personal and sociocultural preferences and values in order to enhance the therapeutic alliance, adherence to treatment, and treatment outcomes. For all these reasons, the APA cautions against the use of guidelines in litigation. Use of these guidelines is voluntary. APA provides the guidelines on an "as is" basis and makes no warranty, expressed or implied, regarding them. APA assumes no responsibility for any injury or damage to persons or property arising out of or related to any use of the guidelines or for any errors or omissions.

The appendices for this guideline, including evidence tables, literature search results, clinical questions, and more, are available online at https://psychiatryonline.org/doi/book/10.1176/appi.books.9780890428023.

Guideline Statement Summary

Assessment and Treatment Planning

1. APA *recommends* **(1C)** that patients with delirium or who are at risk for delirium undergo regular structured assessments for the presence or persistence of delirium using valid and reliable measures.
2. APA *recommends* **(1C)** that a patient's baseline neurocognitive status be determined to permit accurate interpretation of delirium assessments.
3. APA *recommends* **(1C)** that patients with delirium or who are at risk for delirium undergo a detailed review of possible predisposing or contributing factors.
4. APA *recommends* **(1C)** that a detailed medication review be conducted in patients with delirium or who are at risk for delirium, especially those with preexisting cognitive impairment.
5. APA *recommends* **(1C)** that physical restraints not be used in patients with delirium, except in situations when injury to self or others is imminent and only:

    - After review of factors that can contribute to racial/ethnic and other biases in decisions about restraint;
    - With frequent monitoring; and
    - With repeated reassessment of the continued risks and benefits of restraint use as compared with less restrictive interventions.

6. APA *recommends* **(1C)** that patients with delirium have a documented, comprehensive, and person-centered treatment plan.

Nonpharmacological Interventions

7. APA *recommends* **(1B)** that patients with delirium or who are at risk for delirium receive multicomponent nonpharmacological interventions to manage and prevent delirium.

Pharmacological Interventions

8. APA *recommends* **(1C)** that medications, including antipsychotic agents, be used to address neuropsychiatric disturbances of delirium only when all of the following criteria are met:

    - Verbal and nonverbal de-escalation strategies have been ineffective;
    - Contributing factors have been assessed and, as far as possible, addressed; and
    - The disturbances cause the patient significant distress and/or present a risk of physical harm to the patient or others.

9. APA *recommends* **(1C)** that antipsychotic agents not be used to prevent delirium or hasten its resolution.
10. APA *recommends* **(1C)** that benzodiazepines not be used in patients with delirium or who are at risk for delirium, including those with preexisting cognitive impairment, unless there is a specific indication for their use.
11. APA *suggests* **(2B)** that dexmedetomidine be used rather than other sedating agents to prevent delirium in patients who are undergoing major surgery or receiving mechanical ventilation in a critical care setting.
12. APA *suggests* **(2C)** that when patients with delirium are sedated for mechanical ventilation in a critical care setting, dexmedetomidine be used rather than other sedating agents.
13. APA *suggests* **(2C)** that melatonin and ramelteon not be used to prevent or treat delirium.

Transitions of Care

14. APA *recommends* **(1C)** that in patients with delirium or who are at risk for delirium, a detailed medication review, medication reconciliation, and reassessment of the indications for medications, including psychotropic medications, be conducted at transitions of care within the hospital.
15. APA *recommends* **(1C)** that when patients with delirium are transferred to another setting of care, plans for follow-up include:

    - Continued assessments for persistence of delirium;
    - Detailed medication review, medication reconciliation, and reassessment of the indications for medications, including psychotropic medications;
    - Assessment of the consequences of delirium (e.g., posttraumatic symptoms, cognitive impairment); and
    - Psychoeducation about delirium for patients and their care partners.

Guideline Statements and Implementation

Assessment and Treatment Planning

Statement 1 – Structured Assessments for Delirium

APA *recommends* **(1C)** that patients with delirium or who are at risk for delirium undergo regular structured assessments for the presence or persistence of delirium using valid and reliable measures.

Implementation

Patients with delirium often experience a longer and more complicated hospital stay, difficulties in participating in their care, challenges in developing a safe discharge plan, and increased morbidity and mortality (Fong and Inouye 2022; Marcantonio 2017; Prendergast et al. 2022). With early recognition of delirium, potential causes can be identified and addressed, and clinical outcomes can be improved (Devlin et al. 2018). Despite these benefits, delirium is widely known to be underdetected, especially in the acute hospital setting (Bush et al. 2017; Carpenter et al. 2021; Geriatric Medicine Research Collaborative 2019). Research suggests that even highly trained health care professionals may be prone to overlooking delirium in the absence of validated screening tools, underscoring the value of routine assessment for ensuring safe and high-quality care (American College of Surgeons 2019; Bush et al. 2017; Devlin et al. 2007; Grossmann et al. 2014; Kotfis et al. 2018; Spronk et al. 2009). Underrecognition is particularly common among patients with hypoactive delirium (Inouye et al. 2001; van Eijk et al. 2011). Consequently, literature supports the use of regular assessments for monitoring patients for the presence of delirium or exacerbation of symptoms (Bush et al. 2017; Devlin et al. 2018; Kotfis et al. 2018; Mart et al. 2021). The *2018 Clinical Practice Guidelines for the Prevention and Management of Pain, Agitation/Sedation, Delirium, Immobility, and Sleep Disruption in Adult Patients in the ICU* recommend regular assessment of delirium in critical care patients using validated measures (Devlin et al. 2018).

Factors suggesting a need for delirium screening

Use of structured assessments is recommended for patients at risk for delirium as well as in patients who are showing signs of possible delirium. The list of risk factors for delirium is lengthy and includes both predisposing and precipitating factors (Ormseth et al. 2023). Systematic literature reviews and meta-analyses have helped narrow down the list of known risk factors to those with the strongest relationships with delirium. Commonly identified predisposing factors have included, but are not limited to, advanced age, cognitive impairment including dementia and intellectual disability, hearing impairment, functional impairment, multiple comorbidities or frailty, malnutrition, cardiovascular disease, diabetes, central nervous system disorders, depression, and alcohol use disorder (Ormseth et al. 2023; Zaal et al. 2015). Commonly identified precipitating factors have included, but are not limited to, trauma, neurological injury, organ dysfunction (e.g., kidney, liver, respiratory), metabolic abnormalities, hypoalbuminemia, anemia, pain, hypoxemia, fever, infection, medications (e.g., anticholinergics, opioids, benzodiazepines, other sedatives, use of multiple medications), urinary catheterization, and mechanical ventilation (Bramley et al. 2021; Ormseth et al. 2023; Zaal et al. 2015). Among postoperative patients, additional predisposing features include a high score on the American Society of Anesthesiologists (ASA) physical status classification or Charlson Comorbidity Index (Aldecoa et al. 2017; Bramley et al. 2021), whereas additional precipitating factors include the type of surgery, the duration of surgery, the extent of intraoperative blood loss, and the presence of postoperative complications (Aldecoa et al. 2017; Bramley et al. 2021; Ormseth et al. 2023).

The relative contributions of specific risk factors may also vary by treatment setting. For instance, among older adults in the emergency department, delirium was more common in patients who lived in a nursing home (3.4 times more likely), had cognitive impairment (4.4 times more likely), had a hearing impairment (2.5 times more likely), or had a previous stroke (3.2 times more likely) (Oliveira JE Silva et al. 2021). In the postsurgical cardiac setting, being older than 65 was associated with 3 times the risk of developing delirium, having diabetes mellitus with 1.6 times the risk, having cognitive impairment with 5.4 times the risk, and having depression with 3.2 times the risk (Chen et al. 2021). By comparison, in an intensive care unit (ICU) setting, admission risk factors for delirium among individuals age 60 years or older were dementia (odds ratio=6.3), receipt of benzodiazepines before ICU admission (odds ratio=3.4), increased creatinine level (odds ratio=2.1), and low arterial pH (odds ratio=2.1) (Pisani et al. 2007).

General considerations in conducting screening for delirium

In selecting a structured instrument for delirium screening, factors to consider include the availability of the scale (e.g., cost, electronic formats, apps, languages), training and time needed to administer the scale, criteria and population used to validate the scale (e.g., acute vs. long-term care), and sensitivity and specificity of the scale. Scales that are administered on multiple occasions during a hospital or long-term-care stay need to be briefer and require less time to administer than scales that are administered less frequently. The ability to integrate a scale into electronic record systems and day-to-day workflows is also crucial. Furthermore, scales differ in the specific signs and symptoms that they assess. For example, scales such as the Confusion Assessment Method (CAM) will identify stuporous patients as having a possible delirium and will not note whether patients are experiencing psychotic symptoms in the context of delirium. Illusions, hallucinations, and delusions are important to identify because they are often distressing to patients, families, and other caregivers.

In interpreting the results of delirium screening, it is important to recognize that results may be influenced by other conditions that affect a patient's mental state, such as intellectual or developmental disabilities, dementia, catatonia, or severe psychotic or mood disorders. These conditions can also affect measures of delirium severity and will typically lead to false elevations in scores. The timing of delirium screening tool administration is also relevant because a significant fraction of delirious patients will show signs of delirium only at night (Ouimet et al. 2007). In addition, screening should occur when patients have not received sedating medications, if at all possible (van den Boogaard et al. 2020).

Even when validated tools are used to screen for delirium, implementation may be challenging and can affect accurate identification of delirium (Penfold et al. 2024; van Eijk et al. 2011). Thus, concerted efforts are needed to ensure that staff are trained to use delirium screening tools and that the tools are being implemented with fidelity.

Although results of screening tools are helpful, they should not be accepted uncritically. Rather, abnormalities that are detected on screening tools should prompt a more detailed clinical assessment. If screening tests indicate that delirium is present when it is not, unnecessary evaluations could be pursued, including laboratory testing, lumbar puncture, or imaging studies. Conversely, screening tests may fail to detect delirium when it is present. In addition, various screening tools focus on different aspects of delirium and may yield different results. As noted, results may also vary depending on the individual administering the screening tool, the extent of their training and experience, and workflow and staffing considerations (Awan et al. 2021; van Eijk et al. 2011).

Patients' ability to cooperate with screening tool administration can also influence results. A patient's awareness and attention may vary as a result of not only delirium but also other factors such as pain, sedation, or sleep deprivation. The experience of being ill and hospitalized can affect patients' willingness to cooperate with repeated questioning. Some patients may become overstimulated or irritable and refuse to answer questions. In such instances, screening questions may need to be adjusted or postponed.

Structured instruments for delirium screening

Several validated tools stand out as being the most psychometrically sound and in widest use to screen for, diagnose, or assess the severity of delirium. Depending on the patient population, systematic reviews of delirium assessment tools have identified the 4 'A's Test (4AT), Brief CAM (bCAM), CAM, CAM for the Intensive Care Unit (CAM-ICU), 3-minute Diagnostic Interview for the Confusion Assessment Method (3D-CAM), Delirium Diagnostic Tool-Provisional (DDT-Pro), Delirium Observation Screening Scale (DOSS), Delirium Rating Scale—Revised-98 (DRS-R-98), Intensive Care Delirium Screening Checklist (ICDSC), Memorial Delirium Assessment Scale (MDAS), and Nursing Delirium Screening Scale (NuDESC) as having validity, reliability, and/or alignment with DSM-5 diagnostic criteria (Aldwikat et al. 2022; American Psychiatric Association 2013; Gélinas et al. 2018; Helfand et al. 2021; Lin et al. 2023; McCartney et al. 2023; Penfold et al. 2024; Tieges et al. 2021; van Velthuijsen et al. 2016).

To assist in scale selection, features of commonly used scales are described in this section and in Table 2. The Network for Investigation of Delirium: Unifying Scientists website (https://deliriumnetwork.org/measurement) describes several other instruments that can be used to screen for, diagnose, and determine the severity of delirium for clinical or research purposes.

The CAM is a widely used instrument to screen for and diagnose delirium that has been adapted for use in many settings (De and Wand 2015; Wei et al. 2008) and is generally consistent with DSM-5-TR criteria (American Psychiatric Association 2022). Because the CAM has many versions, it is important to be clear about the version being used and whether it has been validated in a given population. Originally, the CAM was studied as a short- and long-form version, with validation based on comparison with delirium criteria in DSM-III-R (American Psychiatric Association 1987). Evidence of delirium on the short-form CAM is indicated by the presence of an acute onset and fluctuating course as well as inattention and either disorganized thinking or altered level of consciousness (Inouye 2014). The long-form CAM includes these four features plus another six that further characterize the mental status. In this guideline, as is common in clinical settings, we use the acronym CAM to refer to the short-form version used for delirium detection. When performed by trained clinicians and scored based on the results of formal cognitive testing, the CAM has reported sensitivities from 94% to 100%, specificities from 90% to 95%, and interrater reliability ranging from 0.81 to 1.00 (Wei et al. 2008).

The CAM-ICU is a structured assessment for scoring the short version of the CAM that was developed specifically for assessing mechanically ventilated patients in the ICU and does not require that patients be verbal. Training is recommended when the CAM-ICU is used, and a training manual is available (Ely 2016). The CAM-ICU consists of the same four core features as the CAM and uses the same scoring algorithm (Ely et al. 2001). The CAM-ICU has excellent sensitivity and specificity, ranging from 95% to 100% and from 93% to 98%, respectively (Wei et al. 2008). The nonverbal items have a sensitivity of 73% and specificity of 100%. The CAM-ICU-7 uses a different scoring approach from the CAM-ICU, with the goal of reflecting delirium severity; scores have

TABLE 2 Summary of validated assessment tools for delirium

Assessment tool	Reference	Number of items	Approximate completion time (minutes)	Advantages	Disadvantages	Access
4AT	MacLullich 2024	4	2	Validated in multiple settings, including acute and long-term care; can be used in nonverbal patients and those who are unable to cooperate with testing; available in 20 languages; can be easily integrated into electronic medical records; no specific training required	Some individual items do not correspond directly to DSM criteria.	Freely available through the 4AT website (https://www.the4at.com/).
bCAM	Han et al. 2013	7	2	Requires minimal training to administer; an algorithmic score calculator available	Available only in English and Zambian; primarily useful for screening; validated primarily in an emergency department setting	The bCAM and its related training materials are freely available on the website of the Vanderbilt University Medical Center for Health Services Research (https://eddelirium.org/delirium-assessment/bcam/).
CAM	Inouye et al. 1990	9	10–15 (long form); 3–5 (short form)	Largely aligns with DSM-5-TR diagnostic criteria; offers two forms (short and long) that incorporate specific cognitive tests as detailed on scoring sheets; can be easily integrated into electronic medical records; can be used for screening, diagnosis, and severity ratings; validated in multiple settings, including acute and long-term care; has been translated into seven languages	The short form does not cover as many domains as some other delirium assessments; thus, the short form may be more reliable as a screening instrument than as a diagnostic one; if used without training, validity and reliability are reduced	The CAM is copyrighted and owned by the American Geriatrics Society. Nonprofit and clinical use are allowed free of charge only after permission is granted from the American Geriatrics Society. Information about obtaining permission can be found at the American Geriatrics Society website (https://www.americangeriatrics.org/about-us/legal-financial-and-government/copyright-permissions).

TABLE 2 Summary of validated assessment tools for delirium (*continued*)

Assessment tool	Reference	Number of items	Approximate completion time (minutes)	Advantages	Disadvantages	Access
CAM-ICU	Ely et al. 2001	9	<5	Requires minimal training to administer; can be used with ventilated and nonverbal patients; can be used for diagnosis; has been translated into 32 languages and validated in 4 languages	Certain items may be difficult to assess in patients with brain injury, cognitive impairment, and moderate to deep sedation.	The CAM-ICU and its related materials (e.g., training materials, pocket guide, worksheets) are freely available for unrestricted use by Vanderbilt University's Critical Illness, Brain Dysfunction, and Survivorship Center. Materials are available in English (https://www.icudelirium.org/medical-professionals/delirium/monitoring-delirium-in-the-icu) and in 31 other languages (https://www.icudelirium.org/medical-professionals/downloads/resource-language-translations).
3D-CAM	Marcantonio et al. 2014	20	2–5	Requires minimal training to administer; can be used for diagnosis; can be scored to reflect delirium severity	May overidentify delirium; requires that patients be able to respond to questions verbally	The 3D-CAM is available in English and 15 other languages (https://americandeliriumsociety.org/ags-cocare-cam-and-help-tools-3d-cam-includes-3d-cam-s-severity/).
DDT-Pro	Kean et al. 2010	3	2	Addresses domains of comprehension, vigilance, and sleep-wake cycle disturbance; two forms are available to reduce practice effects	Requires training of lay raters to administer	Permission to use the DDT-Pro must be obtained from Jose Franco (josefranco11@hotmail.com) or Paula Trzepacz (pttrzepacz@outlook.com); available in English, Japanese, Korean, Spanish, and Thai.

TABLE 2 Summary of validated assessment tools for delirium (*continued*)

Assessment tool	Reference	Number of items	Approximate completion time (minutes)	Advantages	Disadvantages	Access
DRS-R-98	Trzepacz et al. 2001	16	20–30 (scoring), preceded by gathering information from nurses, the family, and the patient chart	Aligns with DSM-5-TR diagnostic criteria; can be used for screening, diagnosis, and severity ratings; has been translated into and validated in six languages	Time-consuming to administer; administration is more labor intensive than some other delirium assessments; designed to be administered by a health care professional with psychiatric training (e.g., psychiatrist, psychologist)	Permission to use the DRS-R-98 must be obtained from the author (Paula Trzepacz; pttrzepacz@outlook.com).
ICDSC	Bergeron et al. 2001	8	7–10	Can be used for screening; can be administered by nonspecialist ICU staff; has been translated to and validated in six languages	May be prone to type I error (false-positive results); not intended to be used for diagnosis or severity ratings	The ICDSC is freely available for clinical or research use; however, the following citation of the original article is required: Bergeron N, Dubois MJ, Dumont M, Dial S, Skrobik Y: "Intensive Care Delirium Screening Checklist: Evaluation of a New Screening Tool." *Intensive Care Medicine* 27(5):859–864, 2001.
MDAS	Breitbart et al. 1997	10	10–15 (scoring), preceded by interviews and gathering information from nurses, the family, and the patient chart	Can be used for severity ratings; well suited for use in delirium treatment research	Not originally designed for use as a screener or diagnostic tool, although data suggest that it can be used as a diagnostic tool as well; does not cover DSM-5 items of acute onset and fluctuating course	The MDAS is freely available from the MDAS publisher's website (https://www.jpsmjournal.com/article/S0885-3924(96)00316-8/pdf).

TABLE 2 Summary of validated assessment tools for delirium (*continued*)

Assessment tool	Reference	Number of items	Approximate completion time (minutes)	Advantages	Disadvantages	Access
NuDESC	Gaudreau et al. 2005	5	<2	Can be used for screening; takes much less time to administer compared with many other validated delirium assessment tools; has been translated into and validated in four languages	Not based on DSM diagnostic criteria and therefore cannot be used for diagnosis; may not be as effective in detecting delirium in hypoactive patients; requires training for administration	The NuDESC is freely available from the NuDESC publisher's website (https://www.jpsmjournal.com/article/S0885-3924(05)00053-9/fulltext).
NH-CAM	Dosa et al. 2007	9	5	Uses existing items from the National Repository of the Minimum Data Set Resident Assessment Instrument for long-term care	Requires training for administration	Uses items B5f, E3, B5a, B5b, B5c, B6, B5d, B5e, and E5 of the National Repository of the Minimum Data Set Resident Assessment Instrument, the full version of which is available at the Centers for Medicare & Medicaid Services website (https://www.cms.gov/medicare/quality/nursing-home-improvement/resident-assessment-instrument-manual).

Note. 4AT=4 'A's Test; bCAM=Brief Confusion Assessment Method; CAM=Confusion Assessment Method; CAM-ICU=Confusion Assessment Method for the Intensive Care Unit; 3D-CAM=3-minute Diagnostic Interview for the Confusion Assessment Method; DDT-Pro=Delirium Diagnostic Tool-Provisional; DRS-R-98=Delirium Rating Scale—Revised-98; DSM=*Diagnostic and Statistical Manual of Mental Disorders*; DSM-5=*Diagnostic and Statistical Manual of Mental Disorders*, 5th Edition; DSM-5-TR=*Diagnostic and Statistical Manual of Mental Disorders*, 5th Edition, Text Revision; ICDSC=Intensive Care Delirium Screening Checklist; ICU=intensive care unit; MDAS=Memorial Delirium Assessment Scale; NH-CAM=Nursing Home Confusion Assessment Method; NuDESC=Nursing Delirium Screening Scale.

Source. Bergeron et al. 2001; Dosa et al. 2007; Gaudreau et al. 2005; Gélinas et al. 2018; Grover and Kate 2012; Helfand et al. 2021; van Velthuijsen et al. 2016.

high internal consistency, good correlations with DRS-R-98 scores, and good predictive validity (Khan et al. 2017; van den Boogaard et al. 2024).

The bCAM is a modified version of the CAM-ICU that was developed for use in settings such as emergency departments, where brevity and sensitivity of screening are of particular importance (Han et al. 2013). The items of the bCAM are rated as being present or absent, and the scale takes less than 2 minutes to complete. Depending on whether the bCAM was completed by a physician or research assistant, the sensitivity and specificity in an emergency department patient population were 78%–84% and 96%–97%, respectively, with good interrater reliability (correlation coefficient kappa=0.88; 95% confidence interval [CI]=0.81–0.95). Training in the use of the bCAM is recommended, and a training manual is available (Han 2015).

The 3D-CAM is a 3-minute diagnostic interview for the CAM that was developed for use in verbal patients (Marcantonio et al. 2014; Palihnich et al. 2023). The authors mapped more than 120 items from the CAM to diagnostic features of delirium and then used item-response theory and statistical approaches to identify 20 of the most informative items. The 3D-CAM shows good agreement with the CAM, although the 3D-CAM may overidentify delirium (Oberhaus et al. 2021). In a sample of medical inpatients older than 75, the 3D-CAM took 2–5 minutes to administer, with a sensitivity of 95% and specificity of 94% for identification of delirium, including hypoactive delirium (Marcantonio et al. 2014). Although the specificity of the 3D-CAM was reduced in individuals with dementia, the sensitivity remained high (Marcantonio et al. 2014). A subsequent systematic review and meta-analysis obtained estimates for pooled positive and negative likelihood ratios of 18.6 and 0.09, respectively (Ma et al. 2023). When an alternative scoring approach is used, the 3D-CAM can be used to assess the severity of delirium as well as its presence (Vasunilashorn et al. 2016). Incorporation of skip logic into the 3D-CAM can further reduce administration times (Marcantonio et al. 2022; Motyl et al. 2020).

For the Ultrabrief CAM (UB-CAM), the clinician asks the patient two questions: months of the year backward and day of the week. If either is answered incorrectly, the other features on the 3D-CAM are assessed. For each feature, remaining questions can be skipped if the patient answers a question incorrectly or if a specific symptom or behavioral observation is present (Fick et al. 2024; Marcantonio et al. 2020). With this approach, available evidence suggests completion times of about 1 minute and sensitivity and specificity values of 93% and 95%, respectively (Motyl et al. 2020).

The Nursing Home CAM (NH-CAM) is derived from the Minimum Data Set Resident Assessment Instrument and contains nine items that cover the same four features as the CAM and CAM-ICU (Dosa et al. 2007; Wei et al. 2008). Scoring is also similar to the CAM and CAM-ICU, but the included algorithms can detect two stages of subsyndromal delirium as well. Although interrater reliability of individual items ranges from 0.38 to 0.80, predictive validity is good, and the NH-CAM can be used to stratify patients on the basis of risk of future rehospitalization and mortality (Dosa et al. 2007).

In addition to the CAM and its different versions, several other delirium scales are relatively brief and have been used to screen for the presence of delirium. The 4AT is named to reflect its four components: Alertness, the Abbreviated Mental Test-4 (AMT4), Attention, and Acute change or fluctuating course (Bellelli et al. 2014). Scores on the 4AT range from 0 to 12, and a value of 4 or greater suggests the possibility of delirium, cognitive impairment, or both (MacLullich 2024). In emergency patients or acute medical patients age 70 or older, the 4AT had a sensitivity of 76% and a specificity of 94% as compared with values of 40% and 100%, respectively, for the CAM relative to a standard assessment using DSM-IV criteria (American Psychiatric Association 1994; Shenkin et al. 2019). A pooled analysis of studies of the 4AT yielded a sensitivity of 88% and a specificity of 88% (Tieges et al. 2021). Elevated scores on the 4AT have been associated with greater rates of mortality (Anand et al. 2022; Evensen et al. 2021).

The NuDESC is a five-item scale that can be quickly administered (generally <2 minutes) to detect delirium (Gaudreau et al. 2005). Items are scored on a scale of 0 to 2, for a total maximum score of 10. A cutoff score of 2 suggests the presence of delirium and has a diagnostic accuracy of 86%. In validation studies, the NuDESC demonstrated a sensitivity of 86% and a specificity of 87% (Gaudreau et al. 2005). Scores on the NuDESC correlated significantly with DSM-IV criteria and with scores from the MDAS.

The ICDSC assesses eight areas on the basis of DSM-IV criteria and common features of delirium (Bergeron et al. 2001). A cutoff score of 4 has been shown to identify delirium in 99% of patients who have the diagnosis but also 36% of patients who do not (Bergeron et al. 2001). Its interrater reliability is high (94%), with an intraclass correlation coefficient of 0.86 (Gélinas et al. 2018). Sensitivity of the ICDSC ranges from 64% to 99%, and specificity ranges from 61% to 88% (Gélinas et al. 2018). In terms of delirium severity, the ICDSC score shows a good correlation with the DRS-98-R score (0.70; 95% CI=0.59–0.79; $P<0.001$; van den Boogaard et al. 2024).

The DDT-Pro includes three items and assesses three core domains of comprehension, vigilance, and sleep-wake cycle disturbance (Kean et al. 2010). Items related to comprehension and vigilance are derived from the Cognitive Test for Delirium (CTD), and the item on sleep-wake cycle disturbance is derived from the DRS-R-98. Each item is scored from 0 to 3 points based on the preceding 12–24 hours. The total score on the DDT-Pro ranges from 0 to 9 points, with 9 being the best performance and 6 or lower serving as a threshold score for a provisional diagnosis of delirium. In a medical inpatient population, the DDT-Pro was noted to have high internal consistency and content validity, as well as good interrater reliability between physicians and nurse administrators and accuracy comparable to that of the CAM (Franco et al. 2020a, 2020b). It also has been tested in skilled nursing facilities, in which about half of the sample had a diagnosis of dementia (Sepúlveda et al. 2021).

Two additional scales provide information on delirium severity and diagnosis. The DRS-R-98 is a 16-item scale rated by clinicians for a 24-hour period, with 13 severity items and 3 diagnostic items, yielding a Total scale (0–46 points) and Severity scale (0–39 points). Higher scores indicate more severe delirium. Validated cutoffs are 18 on the Total scale and 13 on the Severity scale (Trzepacz et al. 2001). The DRS-R-98 provides a detailed phenomenological assessment of delirium that can be used to diagnose and determine the severity of delirium (Trzepacz et al. 2001). Unlike brief screening tools that have been developed for use by nonpsychiatrists, such as the four-item CAM and the 4AT, the DRS-R-98 measures a broad range of delirium symptoms and captures core cognitive, higher-level thinking, and circadian domains of delirium (Franco et al. 2013). It also identifies subsyndromal delirium on the basis of symptoms from these three core domains at milder degrees of item severity (scores 7–12) (Meagher et al. 2014; Sepulveda et al. 2016; Trzepacz et al. 2012). Because the DRS-R-98 uses continuous items that are anchored by phenomenological descriptions of neuropsychiatric symptoms, it is sensitive to change in symptom severity, as demonstrated in longitudinal studies (Leonard et al. 2015) and clinical trials (Trzepacz et al. 2008). Its two motor activity items reflect the motor subtypes of delirium and are validated against the Delirium Motor Subtype Scale and accelerometry (Leonard et al. 2007; Meagher et al. 2008). The DRS-R-98 was originally validated against the CTD, Clinical Global Impression (CGI) scale, and Delirium Rating Scale (DRS), with excellent performance metrics including high validity, reliability, accuracy, internal consistency, and interrater reliability across international samples. Sensitivities ranged from 91% to 100% and specificities from 85% to 100% for the Total score; for Severity scores, sensitivities ranged from 86% to 100% and specificities from 77% to 100%, depending on the cutoffs or comparison groups used. It performs consistently across DSM-III-R, DSM-IV, DSM-5, and ICD-10 diagnostic systems, even with high dementia prevalence (Sepulveda et al. 2015). It does not identify the same patients as having delirium as does the CAM (Meagher et al. 2014; Ryan et al. 2013) and, importantly, does not rate coma as delirium. It is also the only delirium assessment tool validated blindly in a variety of settings and countries against patients with other neuropsychiatric disorders (dementia, depression, mania, schizophrenia) as well as in medical control groups and patients with concomitant dementia (de Negreiros et al. 2008; Franco et al. 2007; Huang et al. 2009; Kato et al. 2010; Lee et al. 2011; Trzepacz et al. 2001).

The MDAS is a 10-item clinician-rated assessment for delirium severity, with scores ranging from 0 to 30 and higher scores indicating greater delirium severity (Breitbart et al. 1997). The MDAS has good interrater reliability (e.g., overall Cronbach's α=0.91), and scores correlate significantly with those from other validated delirium measures, including the DRS, Mini-Mental State Examination (MMSE), and clinician's global rating of delirium and delirium severity. Although the MDAS was not designed as a diagnostic tool, a cutoff score of 13 has been found to adequately discriminate between patients with and without delirium, with a sensitivity of 70% and specificity of 94% (Breitbart et al. 1997).

Although the Richmond Agitation-Sedation Scale (RASS) has been used in some studies, it is not a scale for assessment of delirium. Rather, it is intended for assessing the degree of sedation in critical care patients (Ely et al. 2003). In addition, RASS ratings are centered around 0 and include negative and positive integers. This can yield summary statistics such as mean values that are potentially misleading.

Statement 2 – Determination of Baseline Neurocognitive Status

APA *recommends* **(1C)** that a patient's baseline neurocognitive status be determined to permit accurate interpretation of delirium assessments.

Implementation

To permit accurate interpretation of clinical or structured assessments for delirium, a patient's baseline neurocognitive status should be determined (Duggan et al. 2021; Fong and Inouye 2022; Grover and Kate 2012; Kotfis et al. 2018; Maldonado 2017; Meagher and Leonard 2008; Oh et al. 2017; Ospina et al. 2018). In DSM-5-TR, the criteria for delirium require that "the disturbance ... represents a change from baseline attention and awareness" (American Psychiatric Association 2022, p. 672). Accordingly, many screening tools for delirium also incorporate a requirement that the patient's clinical findings must represent a change from their baseline cognitive functioning.

Baseline neurocognitive status is also essential to determining when delirium has resolved. The longitudinal course of delirium varies, but delirium still may be present when a patient leaves the hospital and for some time thereafter (Pereira et al. 2021; Wilcox et al. 2021). Obtaining and documenting the patient's baseline neurocognitive status at the time of index hospitalization will reduce the confounding effects of retrospective recall and will aid in identifying persistent delirium.

Baseline neurocognitive status can be determined in several ways. For patients who are being admitted for an elective surgical procedure (e.g., major orthopedic or cardiac surgery) that is associated with a significant risk of delirium, administering a cognitive screening test such as the Montreal Cognitive Assessment (MoCA; Nasreddine et al. 2005) in advance of the procedure may be helpful. In other circumstances, information can be obtained by speaking with family members or others who are part of the patient's support network. Although developed for use in assessing individuals with dementia, tools such as the Informant Questionnaire on Cognitive Decline in the Elderly (IQCODE; Burton et al. 2021b, 2021c; Jorm 1994; Jorm and Jacomb 1989) or the Ascertain Dementia 8 (AD-8; Galvin et al. 2005; Tanwani et al. 2023) can be completed by an informant and may be helpful in identifying whether a patient with delirium had preexisting cognitive impairment. Review of past medical records and input from the patient's primary care clinician can also provide details on the patient's baseline cognitive status. Even if no specific information is available on the patient's earlier cognition, knowledge of the patient's previous functioning, such as academic or employment status, and their level of education may be helpful in identifying likely changes from baseline. In individuals with intellectual or developmental disabilities, knowledge of baseline neurocognitive status is particularly important in assessing for delirium (Simpson 2003; Van Waarde and Van Der Mast 2004). Determining baseline neurocognitive status can also be a challenge in individuals with preexisting cognitive impairment related to conditions such as stroke, traumatic brain injury, dementia, or other degenerative nervous system disease (Fong and Inouye 2022; Stroomer-van Wijk et al. 2016; Zeilinger et al. 2022).

Rates of preexisting cognitive impairment are increased in hospitalized patients (Halladay et al. 2018; Peel et al. 2019). In ICU settings, the prevalence of preexisting cognitive impairment has been reported to be 37% among patients age 65 years and older (Pisani et al. 2003). Individuals with preexisting cognitive impairment may be more likely to develop delirium during a hospital stay, and knowledge of baseline cognitive status may help in determining relative risk (Halladay et al. 2018; Tsui et al. 2022; Zipser et al. 2021). Such individuals also may have more difficulty providing information on delirium symptoms or factors such as pain that can contribute to delirium. In addition, cognitive changes that do occur may be erroneously disregarded by clinicians if they are viewed as a manifestation of the patient's baseline cognitive impairment (Bergl 2019; Oh et al. 2017; The Joint Commission 2022). Interventions that are aimed at reducing or preventing delirium, such as orienting the patient or providing education, also may require adjustment if a patient has a preexisting cognitive impairment.

Statement 3 – Review for Predisposing or Contributing Factors

APA *recommends* **(1C)** that patients with delirium or who are at risk for delirium undergo a detailed review of possible predisposing or contributing factors.

Implementation

As discussed in Statement 1, multiple factors can predispose to or contribute to the development of delirium, although risk factors (as shown in Table 3) may differ with the patient population, treatment setting, or subtype of delirium (Aldecoa et al. 2017; Bramley et al. 2021; Ghezzi et al. 2022; Krewulak et al. 2020; Ormseth et al. 2023; Wilson et al. 2020; Zaal et al. 2015). Individuals also may have several of these factors that together contribute to the development of delirium, although each factor alone may not have precipitated a delirious state. Because delirium is not a unitary entity with a single cause, it is only through addressing these manifold precipitating and predisposing factors, insofar as possible, that we can fully treat delirium in individual patients.

An increase in delirium risk has also been noted in the literature with factors that likely act in a complex or indirect fashion (e.g., recent fall; hip fracture; trauma; hospitalization; ICU admission; specific surgical procedures; hospital-acquired conditions; use of interventions that restrict movement such as cardiac monitoring, intravenous lines, traction device, or pneumatic leg compression devices). Other factors may worsen the apparent symptoms of delirium. For example, an individual who is restrained, in pain, or withdrawing from nicotine may become more agitated if they have delirium, or an individual whose primary language differs from that of the staff may be less likely to receive interventions such as frequent reorientation. These factors are also important to recognize in providing quality care to patients with delirium.

The presence of neurocognitive impairment, including intellectual disability and dementia, is a frequent predisposing factor in individuals who develop delirium and may change the interpretation of cognitive findings (Fong and Inouye 2022; Fong et al. 2015, 2022; Halladay et al. 2018; National Task Group on Intellectual Disabilities and Dementia Practices and the Health Matters Program 2023; Tsui et al. 2022; Zipser et al. 2021). In hospitalized patients, it has been estimated that up to half of the individuals with dementia will also have superimposed delirium (Han et al. 2022).

Table 3 Some common predisposing and contributing factors to delirium

Demographic factors

Advancing age, commonly defined as 65 years or older

Residing in structured setting (e.g., residential, long-term care)

Aspects of history

Prior delirium

Co-occurring conditions

Psychiatric disorders

- Cognitive impairment, including prior dementia
- Alcohol or other substance use disorders
- Depressive disorders

Other central nervous system abnormalities

- Cerebrovascular disease, including stroke
- Alzheimer's disease
- Parkinson's disease
- Traumatic brain injury
- Meningitis or encephalitis
- Vasculitis
- Seizure disorder
- Other central nervous system disorders

Other medical illnesses

- Infection (e.g., pneumonia, urinary tract infection, HIV, COVID-19)
- Sepsis
- Cardiovascular disease (e.g., heart failure)
- Pulmonary disease (e.g., chronic obstructive pulmonary disease)
- Kidney disease
- Hepatic failure
- Diabetes mellitus
- Other endocrine abnormalities (e.g., thyroid, adrenal)
- Metastatic disease
- Paraneoplastic syndromes
- Obstructive sleep apnea
- Multiple chronic conditions, including as measured by Charlson Comorbidity Index

Commonly implicated medications and other substances

Specific medications and medication classes

- Benzodiazepine or other sedatives
- Medications with anticholinergic properties

Table 3 Some common predisposing and contributing factors to delirium (*continued*)

- Opioid analgesics, including meperidine
- Corticosteroids
- Immunosuppressive agents
- Sympathomimetics

Misused or abused substances (e.g., synthetic cannabinoids, alcohol, cocaine, opioids, sedative-hypnotics, stimulants, psychedelics)

Herbal medications or nutraceuticals

Use of multiple medications, including adding three or more medications during admission

Medication-related toxicities

- Neuroleptic malignant syndrome
- Serotonin syndrome
- Toxicity with elevated serum levels (e.g., lithium, valproic acid, carbamazepine, amiodarone, digoxin, phenytoin, salicylate)
- Medication-related metabolic disturbances (e.g., hyponatremia related to antidepressants or carbamazepine, hyperammonemia related to valproic acid)

Toxins (e.g., heavy metals, pesticides, solvents, carbon monoxide)

Physiological abnormalities

Hypotension

Anemia or significant blood loss, including situations requiring blood transfusions

Metabolic disturbances (e.g., sodium, calcium, magnesium, phosphate abnormalities)

Acid-base abnormalities

Hyperammonemia

Hypoglycemia

Elevated blood urea nitrogen (BUN)/creatinine

Hypoxemia

Malnutrition or hypoalbuminemia

Vitamin deficiency (e.g., thiamine, vitamin B_6, vitamin B_{12})

Sensory or functional impairments

Visual impairment

Hearing impairment

Immobility

Frailty[a]

Other functional impairments

Factors related to urgent/emergent procedures

High ASA status

Recent surgical complications, including cardiopulmonary complications

Operative times

TABLE 3 Some common predisposing and contributing factors to delirium (*continued*)
Factors related to urgent/emergent procedures (*continued*)
Anesthesia type and depth
Prolonged time on cardiac bypass
Factors related to hospitalization
High illness severity (e.g., as reflected by an elevated APACHE score or SOFA score)
Use of indwelling bladder catheter
Use of mechanical ventilation
Other factors
Fever
Dehydration
Constipation, including fecal impaction
Urinary retention
New pressure ulcers
Hyper- or hypothermia
Sleep deprivation or sleep-wake cycle disturbance
Social isolation
Lack of a familiar environment
Environmental overstimulation

Note. APACHE=Acute Physiology and Chronic Health Evaluation; ASA=American Society of Anesthesiologists; COVID-19=coronavirus SARS-CoV-2 disease 2019; HIV=human immunodeficiency virus; SOFA=Sequential Organ Failure Assessment.

[a]Examples of scales that have been used to assess frailty include, but are not limited to, the Cardiovascular Health Study Index, also referred to as Fried's frailty phenotype; the Clinical Frailty Scale; the Edmonton Frailty Scale; the Fatigue, Resistance, Ambulation, Illness, and Loss of Weight Index (FRAIL); and the Frailty Index of Accumulated Deficits of Rockwood and Mitnitski.

Source. Ali et al. 2021; Béland et al. 2021; Bramley et al. 2021; Bush and Bruera 2009; Chaiwat et al. 2019; Chen et al. 2021; Duceppe et al. 2019; Featherstone et al. 2022; Fong et al. 2015; Geriatric Medicine Research Collaborative 2019; Girard et al. 2018; Greaves et al. 2020; Hshieh et al. 2020; Iamaroon et al. 2020; Kang et al. 2019; Maldonado 2017; Marquetand et al. 2021, 2022; Mattison 2020; Mauri et al. 2021; Mevorach et al. 2023; Nagari and Babu 2019; Oliveira JE Silva et al. 2021; Ormseth et al. 2023; Pisani et al. 2007; Pun et al. 2021; Saljuqi et al. 2020; Spiropoulou et al. 2022; Vacas et al. 2022; Visser et al. 2021; Wilke et al. 2022; Wilson et al. 2020; Zaal et al. 2015; Zhang et al. 2021; Zipser et al. 2019a, 2019b.

Substantial rates of delirium superimposed on dementia are also found in other settings of care, although there is a high degree of variability in reported rates depending on the patient population and rating approach (de Lange et al. 2013; Fick et al. 2002; Morandi et al. 2012, 2014). As described in Statement 2, this makes it important to determine the patient's baseline neurocognitive status, to identify whether cognitive impairment is present prior to hospitalization, and to determine whether patients have delirium alone or delirium superimposed on preexisting cognitive impairment. Patients who are frail have a high rate of developing delirium, but paradoxically, delirium is less likely to be identified when patients are frail (Geriatric Medicine Research Collaborative 2019). Although biases in the diagnosis of delirium are not well studied, incorrect assumptions about decline or fluctuation in cognition in older individuals may play a role. Biases also exist toward individuals with disabilities that may affect recognition of delirium (Johnston et al. 2022; Lagu et al. 2022). In addition, racial or ethnic biases may influence the identification of delirium or associated risk factors for delirium. For example, one study showed that Black individuals were more likely than other patients to be identified as cognitively impaired, independent of actual results on a cognitive screening test (Campbell et al. 2014). For these reasons, it is crucial to consider the effect of possible biases in diagnosing delirium or identifying predisposing or contributing factors to delirium.

Although a substantial number of risk factors appear to be associated with an increase in the likelihood of delirium, many individuals who have these factors will not have delirium. Possible precipitants or contributors to delirium also need to be considered in the context of other clinical findings. For example, a female may have evidence of bacteriuria due to urinary colonization without having it precipitate or contribute to delirium (Krinitski et al. 2021; Nicolle 2016; Nicolle et al. 2019). Thus, it would be important to determine whether the patient has other urinary symptoms or signs of systemic infection, such as fever or an elevated white blood cell count (Krinitski et al. 2021; Nicolle 2016; Nicolle et al. 2019). Other sources of infection also would need to be ruled out before attributing delirium to a urinary tract infection. Without a detailed consideration of the meaning of a finding such as bacteriuria, antibiotics may contribute to delirium (Bhattacharyya et al. 2016), be instituted inappropriately and contribute to antibiotic resistance, or target the wrong organism and be ineffective (Nicolle 2016; Nicolle et al. 2019).

Information about possible predisposing or contributing factors might be obtained from patients who are able to respond to questions or from family members or others involved in the patient's care. Other physicians or health care professionals who are treating the patient can be contacted for information, and details of medical history, prior cognitive or functional status, current problems, and medications may be available through medical records, prescription monitoring data programs (PMDPs), external prescribing histories, health information exchanges (HIEs), and other electronic sources of information. Patients or families also may be able to bring in current prescription bottles to determine current medication regimens.

Additional health-related information will become available in the course of evaluation through physical examination, laboratory studies, or other tests (e.g., imaging, electrocardiography, cultures). No routine battery of tests or other investigations should be done in all patients with delirium or who are at risk for delirium. Rather, the evaluation will depend on careful review of the available information to identify common contributors to delirium and factors of relevance to the individual patient's condition, and additional history or testing should be obtained as clinically indicated (Table 4).

TABLE 4 **Suggested laboratory tests and other studies in the assessment of patients with delirium**
Commonly done laboratory tests and other studies
Vital signs (pulse rate, blood pressure, respiratory rate, temperature; orthostatic pulse and blood pressure if indicated)
Pulse oximetry
Complete blood count with differential
Glucose measurement
Comprehensive metabolic panel
Urinalysis
Laboratory tests and studies that are sometimes done, depending on history, clinical findings, and results of other evaluations
Magnesium level
Phosphate level
Creatine phosphokinase (CPK)[a] level
Ammonia level
Thyroid-stimulating hormone (TSH) level

TABLE 4 Suggested laboratory tests and other studies in the assessment of patients with delirium (*continued*)

Laboratory tests and studies that are sometimes done, depending on history, clinical findings, and results of other evaluations (*continued*)
Vitamin B_{12}; methylmalonic acid level, as indicated
Thiamine level
Serum levels of medications (e.g., lithium, valproic acid, carbamazepine, amiodarone, digoxin, phenytoin, salicylate)
C-reactive protein and/or erythrocyte sedimentation rate (ESR)
Antinuclear antibody (ANA) level
Severe coronavirus SARS-CoV-2 disease 2019 (COVID-19) test
Human immunodeficiency virus (HIV) test
Syphilis test[b]
Blood gases
Cultures (e.g., urine, blood, sputum, wound, cerebrospinal fluid)
Blood alcohol level
Urinary toxicology screen, with confirmation if appropriate
Bladder scan[c]
Abdominal X-ray: kidney, ureter, and bladder (KUB) view
Chest X-ray
Neuroimaging (e.g., brain magnetic resonance imaging, head computed tomography)[d]
Electroencephalogram
Lumbar puncture[e]

[a]Significant elevations of CPK can be seen in neuroleptic malignant syndrome or serotonin syndrome.

[b]Under most circumstances, it is recommended to screen with an initial nontreponemal test (e.g., Venereal Disease Research Laboratory or rapid plasma reagin test) with confirmation of a positive result using a treponemal antibody detection test (e.g., *Treponema pallidum* particle agglutination test) (U.S. Preventive Services Task Force 2022).

[c]Obtain to identify urinary retention.

[d]Although neuroimaging is often done in patients with delirium and no recent head trauma, clinically significant findings are uncommon in the absence of focal neurological findings (Butcher et al. 2023; Finkelmeier et al. 2019; S. Lee et al. 2023; Liu et al. 2023; Theisen-Toupal et al. 2014).

[e]Consultation with neurology is suggested prior to lumbar puncture to determine the most appropriate tests to obtain on the cerebrospinal fluid.

Statement 4 – Review of Medications

APA *recommends* **(1C)** that a detailed medication review be conducted in patients with delirium or who are at risk for delirium, especially those with preexisting cognitive impairment.

Implementation

As discussed in Statement 3 and delineated in Table 3, several medications and medication classes may contribute to delirium. Individuals with preexisting cognitive impairment are often sensitive to the effects of such medications. Consequently, in patients who have delirium or who are at risk for delirium (as described in Statements 1 and 3), a detailed review of medications is helpful. The goals of a detailed medication review include obtaining an accurate list of the patient's medications. In addition to identifying medications that have a significant likelihood of contributing to delirium, other goals of medication review include identifying agents that could be reduced in dose, that may no longer be needed, or that may be contributing to drug-drug or drug-disease interactions. It is also important to note any recent changes in the doses of medications or over-the-counter products and whether medications or over-the-counter products have recently been started or stopped, intentionally or inadvertently.

Much has been written about approaches to obtaining a medication history and clarifying discrepancies in the medication list, a process known as *medication reconciliation* (Greenwald et al. 2010; Schnipper et al. 2022). For patients who are admitted from another facility, a current medication list typically will be provided. In other circumstances, information sources that can be used in constructing the medication list include interviewing the patient, the patient's family, and other involved caregivers; asking to see the patient's medication bottles; accessing recent records through an electronic health record (EHR) or HIE; accessing recent pharmacy dispensing records through external pharmacy prescribing databases; or checking PMDPs for histories of controlled substance prescriptions (Centers for Disease Control and Prevention 2021). The complete medication list should include prescribed medications as well as over-the-counter medications, herbal products, supplements, or nutraceuticals whether taken on a routine or "as-needed" (i.e., prn) basis. The dose, route, frequency, and indication for the medication should be listed when known. Documenting the date and time of the last medication dose is also helpful when scheduling and informing patients about the timing of next doses at transitions of care.

Although medication reconciliation has been recommended for use at transitions of care and in ambulatory settings for more than a decade, there are still challenges in its application and limitations in the evidence supporting its use (Ceschi et al. 2021; Killin et al. 2021; Mekonnen et al. 2016a; Redmond et al. 2018; Rungvivatjarus et al. 2020; Tamblyn et al. 2019). Patients, family members, or other involved caregivers may not have access to current medications in the context of an emergency visit or hospital admission. Follow-up is often needed to complete the initial medication history. Prescribed medications may have changed since the patient's last visit to a facility, or they may not have been taking a medication even though it was dispensed by a pharmacy or recorded in a PMDP. When patients are taking long-acting medications (e.g., long-acting injectable formulations of antipsychotic medications, naltrexone, or contraceptives; implantable formulations of contraceptives), EHRs may not list them as active medications, and patients or other informants may not recall that they are taking them unless specifically asked. For medications that are prescribed on an as-needed (i.e., prn) basis, the frequency of actual use may be quite variable. It can be difficult to obtain a full list of over-the-counter medications, herbal products, supplements, and nutraceuticals, and these may include contaminants and may vary in their active ingredients or medication interactions, even when they are documented.

As a result of the complexities of medication reconciliation, errors of omission may occur in taking the medication history. Also, medications that have been previously discontinued may be erroneously resumed as part of the medication reconciliation process. With medications that require gradual dose adjustment on initiation (e.g., clozapine, lamotrigine), an abrupt resumption of a therapeutic dose of medication can lead to adverse effects.

Evidence suggests that the medication reconciliation process can be more efficient and more effective when done by a pharmacist, pharmacy technician, or other designated staff member who has knowledge of medications (Marshall et al. 2022; Mekonnen et al. 2016b; Schnipper et al. 2023). Such an approach is now required in acute care settings in some jurisdictions (California Senate Bill No. 1254 2018). Without a designated individual to be responsible for medication reconciliation, accountability is unclear, and in a busy clinical environment, obtaining the medication history may be delayed or bypassed entirely.

Once the medication list has been documented as accurately as possible, review of the medication list can determine whether specific medications can be reduced in dose or discontinued, a process that has been termed *deprescribing* (Bloomfield et al. 2020; Curtin et al. 2020; Lee et al. 2021;

McDonald et al. 2022; Reeve 2020). As discussed in Statement 3, medications that may be more likely to contribute to delirium include benzodiazepines or other sedatives, narcotic analgesics, corticosteroids, sympathomimetic agents, and medications with anticholinergic properties (Maldonado 2017; Mattison 2020; Ryan and Kimchi 2021). Delirium also may occur in the context of medication-related toxicity syndromes (e.g., neuroleptic malignant syndrome [NMS], serotonin syndrome) or with elevated serum levels of medications (e.g., lithium, valproic acid, carbamazepine, amiodarone, digoxin, phenytoin, salicylate). Medication-specific effects, such as hyperammonemia due to valproic acid or hyponatremia due to antidepressive agents, also should be considered. Many tools are available to help identify other medications that may need to be tapered or discontinued (Reeve 2020), but the Beers Criteria (American Geriatrics Society Beers Criteria® Update Expert Panel 2023) and the STOPP/START criteria (O'Mahony et al. 2015) are commonly referenced.

Pharmacokinetic and pharmacodynamic considerations are also relevant when reviewing medications (Derendorf and Schmidt 2020; Levenson and Ferrando 2024), identifying those that may be contributing to delirium, and determining when tapering or discontinuation of a medication may be indicated. When a patient is prescribed multiple medications, it is always helpful to use a medication interaction database to determine whether drug-drug interactions may be occurring. Such interactions can be mediated by metabolic enzymes (e.g., cytochrome P450 [CYP] enzyme system), drug transporters (e.g., P-glycoprotein), displacement from protein binding sites, or other mechanisms (Akamine et al. 2012; Armstrong et al. 2003; Darwich and von Moltke 2019; Derendorf and Schmidt 2020; Flockhart et al. 2021; Gessner et al. 2019; Kiang et al. 2005; Levenson and Ferrando 2024; Linnet and Ejsing 2008; Sandson et al. 2005; Tornio et al. 2019). In other circumstances, medication side effects, such as sedation or hypotension, may be additive or synergistic when associated with two or more medications. Medication absorption and first-pass metabolism of medications may be altered by disease (e.g., bowel disease; Megna and Vaughn 2022), prior surgical procedures (e.g., bariatric surgery, gastric or intestinal resection; Brill et al. 2015; Roerig and Steffen 2015), or other medications (e.g., those that affect gastrointestinal pH, transit times, microbiome, or bile acid synthesis; Demeester et al. 2023). Other pharmacokinetic factors that can influence medication levels include age, body size, relative body fat, genetic subtypes of metabolic enzymes (e.g., rapid vs. slow metabolizer status), and renal and hepatic status (Derendorf and Schmidt 2020; Gouju and Legeay 2023; Keller and Hann 2018; Levenson and Ferrando 2024; Mangoni and Jackson 2004; Trifirò and Spina 2011). Medications that are lipophilic will be distributed in greater levels to body fat and to the brain. As a result, when levels of lipophilic medications have been high, delirium and other central nervous system findings may dissipate gradually after medication tapering or discontinuation. Pharmacodynamic considerations that may affect medication responses or side effects in the aging brain include neurotransmitter and receptor changes (e.g., cholinergic, dopaminergic) (Mangoni and Jackson 2004; Trifirò and Spina 2011).

As with any decisions related to medications, it is important for the members of the health care team to consider the potential benefits, side effects, and other disadvantages of a medication before adjusting a medication dose. When a medication is effective and well tolerated, it will generally be continued; however, in some circumstances, pharmacokinetic considerations or other factors may make it preferable to change to another medication in the same class. In other circumstances, an effort may be made to reduce the dose of a medication, particularly when it is known to contribute to delirium or to other potential adverse effects, such as falls. When a medication is usually not effective in a specific condition or is otherwise not needed (e.g., some over-the-counter products, herbal preparations, supplements), tapering and discontinuation may be most appropriate.

Even when tapering or discontinuing a medication seems indicated, it is important to make such decisions in the context of patient-centered decision-making when the patient is able to participate or in discussion with the patient's health care designee. Individuals, their family members, or other caregivers may be fearful or ambivalent about tapering specific medications because of negative experiences with deprescribing or severe symptoms that seemed to be controlled by the current regimen (Sawan et al. 2020; Scott et al. 2022). Individuals may also view deprescribing as an indication that their care is being reduced because of costs, biases, or clinician disengagement (Sawan et al. 2020; Scott et al. 2022). Thus, it is important to obtain patient, family member, and caregiver perspectives and provide information on the reasons for deprescribing whenever possible.

When a patient has been taking a stable dose of medication for some time, abrupt tapering or discontinuation could destabilize an underlying condition or result in a withdrawal syndrome (e.g., with sedatives, opioids, some antidepressants). Patients who are receiving a high dose of medication or have had a lengthy period of treatment will typically need a slower speed of medication tapering than individuals taking lower medication doses for a shorter period (Pottie et al. 2018). In assessing the effects of medication reduction or discontinuation, it also may be preferable to make changes gradually, if possible, so that emergent symptoms or other effects of dose adjustment can be interpreted. Factors such as medication half-life or the presence of long-half-life active metabolites are also relevant to interpreting the effects of medication tapering or discontinuation (Hendset et al. 2006).

Statement 5 – Use of Restraints

APA *recommends* **(1C)** that physical restraints not be used in patients with delirium, except in situations when injury to self or others is imminent and only:

- After review of factors that can contribute to racial/ethnic and other biases in decisions about restraint;
- With frequent monitoring; and
- With repeated reassessment of the continued risks and benefits of restraint use as compared with less restrictive interventions.

Implementation

Use of physical restraints should be minimized and limited to situations when injury to self or others is imminent. Physical restraint use may be associated with several potential harms, including pressure ulcers, fractures, cardiac arrhythmias, musculoskeletal injuries, deep vein thrombosis, aspiration pneumonia, worsening of agitation, and, in rare instances, asphyxiation with potential death from strangulation (Berzlanovich et al. 2012; Ertuğrul and Özden 2020; Funayama and Takata 2020; Sharifi et al. 2021; Teece et al. 2020). These risks may be greater in individuals with impaired consciousness, as occurs in patients with delirium, or in patients with existing conditions such as musculoskeletal or cardiorespiratory disease. Psychologically, use of physical restraints is often distressing to patients and families (American Psychiatric Association 2022; Perez et al. 2022; Sharifi et al. 2021; Smithard and Randhawa 2022; Wong et al. 2020). It is important to be aware of the patient's experiences, such as a history of trauma or prior physical restraint, that would add to the distress of being restrained while delirious. Posttraumatic stress disorder (PTSD) may also occur in individuals who have been physically restrained, although it is unclear whether the risk is due to restraints, per se, or is related to other aspects of receiving care for critical illness (Franks et al. 2021; Hatchett et al. 2010; Jones et al. 2007; Zghidi et al. 2019). Consequently, before deciding to use physical restraints, it is essential to weigh these risks against the intended benefits of restraint use as compared with other possible interventions.

Often, physical restraints are considered in an effort to enhance patient safety, prevent self-extubation or tube dislodgment, reduce the risk of falls, or protect staff from patient combativeness (Devlin et al. 2018). However, the few studies that have examined these outcomes have not shown a reduction in these risks with the use of physical restraints (Perez et al. 2019; Rose et al. 2016). Thus, except in an urgent or emergent situation, other interventions typically should be attempted before initiating physical restraints (American Psychiatric Association 2022; Knox and Holloman 2012; Roppolo et al. 2020). In addition, efforts should be made to treat underlying contributors to delirium (see Statement 3) or other factors that may be affecting agitation, such as pain or co-occurring psychiatric conditions.

Attention to the safety of the patient and others should always be a top priority. This may involve repositioning equipment or moving objects from the bedside that could be used to harm self or others. Environmental modifications can be attempted to promote a more calming environment (e.g., turning off the television, providing a single room). To reduce agitation, issues of comfort also should be addressed, such as pain, environmental temperature, urinary retention, constipation, hunger, thirst, positioning in bed, and constraints of monitoring leads or catheters. It also may be possible to reduce restraint use through nonpharmacological approaches such as educating family members and involving them in the care plan or having a staff member sit with the patient to provide redirection and reassurance (Cui et al. 2022). Verbal de-escalation techniques are often suggested as a way to help patients calm themselves (American Psychiatric Association 2022; Knox and Holloman 2012; Richmond et al. 2012; Roppolo et al. 2020); however, this approach may not be as effective with patients who are delirious and unable to attend to or process verbal communication. If verbal de-escalation is used, it is important to be respectful, listen to what the patient is saying, use a soft voice, be concise, and set appropriate limits without being provocative (Roppolo et al. 2020). Medication, if used judiciously, can also be helpful in calming the patient (see Statements 8, 9, and 10) and may help in avoiding the use of restraint or reducing its duration. In addition, receiving medication is less distressing to most patients than being physically restrained.

If physical restraint is being considered to address the safety of the patient or others, it is important to be aware of biases that may influence decision-making. For example, implicit biases about race, ethnicity, or other factors may be accentuated when clinicians are stressed, fatigued, or under pressure to make a rapid decision (Agboola et al. 2021; Johnson et al. 2016). Thus, it is important for clinicians and organizations to be aware of national recommendations for the provision of culturally and linguistically appropriate services and make consistent efforts to reduce associated health disparities (Centers for Medicare & Medicaid Services 2016).

Minimal information is available on biases that affect restraint-related decision-making in patients with delirium. However, a U.S. sample of all acute care hospital discharges found that 7.4% of patients with a diagnosis of "encephalitis" were restrained and that Black patients were more likely to be physically restrained than White patients (Luccarelli et al. 2023). In a subset of the sample who had dementia with a behavioral disturbance, a disproportionately higher percentage of Black patients was found among the individuals who were physically restrained during admission (Singh et al. 2023). Similarly, in emergency department encounters, including those for emergency psychiatric evaluations, most (Carreras Tartak et al. 2021; Schnitzer et al. 2020; C.M. Smith et al. 2022; Walia et al. 2023; Wong et al. 2021), but not all (Conteh et al. 2024), studies have shown a significantly greater likelihood of being physically restrained in Black patients compared with White patients. Some (Khatri et al. 2022; Robinson et al. 2022), but not all (Conteh et al. 2024; Wong et al. 2021), studies have shown that Black patients also were more likely to be given sedating medications (e.g., antipsychotics, benzodiazepines, ketamine) to address agitation in emergency settings. Information on the relative likelihood of physical restraint among Asian patients or Hispanic patients has been mixed, with some studies showing greater restraint rates and other studies showing lower or similar restraint rates compared with those in White patients (Carreras Tartak et al. 2021; Conteh et al. 2024; Schnitzer et al. 2020; Walia et al. 2023; Wong et al. 2021). In a Canadian study of patients with delirium, a significantly greater rate of physical restraint use was reported among patients who did not prefer English as their dominant language compared with patients who did prefer English (Reppas-Rindlisbacher et al. 2022). Furthermore, men consistently had greater restraint rates than women, but no data were reported for individuals of other genders (Schnitzer et al. 2020; Walia et al. 2023; Wong et al. 2021).

It is important to note that some approaches that have been developed to assist staff in addressing behavioral issues may also show racial biases. These could, in turn, influence and interject systemic biases into decisions about restraint. For example, one approach to managing behavioral issues in hospital inpatients on nonpsychiatric services has been to deploy behavioral response teams. Although the efficacy of such teams has not been well studied, one report suggests that a behavioral response team at one hospital was contacted more often about Black patients than about White patients (Moore et al. 2019). Another study of a behavioral response team found that Black and Asian patients were more likely to receive parenteral medications, and a numerically greater percentage of Black patients were placed in four-point restraints as compared with other racial or ethnic groups (Caravella et al. 2023). In terms of emergency security responses, rates were significantly higher in Black than in White patients, whereas rates for Hispanic and non-Hispanic patients did not differ (Valtis et al. 2023). Electronic behavioral alerts are an additional method that has been used to alert staff to patients who had safety-related concerns on a previous visit, typically verbal or physical incidents involving other patients or staff members. Here too, non-Hispanic Black patients were substantially more likely to have an electronic behavioral alert on their chart than non-Hispanic White patients, and men were more likely to have such an alert than women (Haimovich et al. 2024). Thus, if electronic behavioral alerts are used, it is important to institute processes for reviewing them for possible bias and linking them to patient-specific plans of care for addressing behavioral issues.

If physical restraint is still believed to be indicated after considering the risks and benefits of restraint, use of other interventions, and sources of potential bias in decision-making, the type of restraint chosen should be targeted to the patient's circumstances and be as minimally restrictive as possible. For example, the use of mittens may prevent a patient from pulling at tubes without being as restrictive to patient movement as soft limb restraints. The duration of restraint should be as brief as possible, and repeated reassessments of patients' status are essential, particularly given the waxing and waning nature of delirium.

It is also critical to monitor the patient closely while physical restraints are in place. The specific monitoring requirements will be determined by the requirements of the Centers for Medicare & Medicaid Services (CMS) Conditions of Participation (Code of Federal Regulations 2023), The Joint Commission or other accrediting bodies, state regulations, and hospital policy. However, monitoring should include physiological monitoring (e.g., vital signs, evidence of circulatory or neuronal impairments in extremities with limb restraints), assessment of psychological symptoms in response to restraints, and attention to nutrition, hydration, or elimination needs while restrained. Respect for the patient's privacy while in restraints is also crucial. Once the period of restraint has ended, it is helpful to discuss the experience with patients who are able and with family members or others who are part of the patient's care team to address any questions or concerns related to the restraint episode.

Statement 6 – Person-Centered Treatment Planning

APA *recommends* **(1C)** that patients with delirium have a documented, comprehensive, and person-centered treatment plan.

Implementation

No single medication or intervention serves as a universal treatment for all patients with delirium. Rather, treatment is individualized based on the patient's clinical picture. Delirium has multiple etiologies, heterogeneous phenotypes, and numerous potential risk factors (see Statement 3); thus, treatment planning may be challenging, and changes in the treatment plan are often needed (Devlin et al. 2018; Mart et al. 2021; Ormseth et al. 2023). Individuals who are older, are frail, or have significant multisystem disease may have limited reserves and less resilience in the face of physiological disruptions, a situation that has been termed *homeostenosis* (Fried et al. 2021). Consequently, factors, combinations of factors, or degrees of abnormality may be overlooked or de-emphasized as being unlikely to cause delirium in individuals with greater reserves. Decision-making also may be influenced by biases related to apparent functioning at baseline (Bergl 2019) or related to race, ethnicity, gender, or age (see Statement 5). Thorough documentation of a comprehensive, person-centered treatment plan reduces the possibility of biases and helps ensure that interventions are appropriately selected to fit the clinical setting and address the full range of each patient's medical and psychosocial needs (Table 5).

TABLE 5 Factors to consider in developing a person-centered treatment plan

Medical interventions, including medication review

- Instituting specific interventions to address likely contributors to the patient's delirium (see Statement 3), recognizing that multiple contributors may coexist
- Reviewing and, if indicated, adjusting medications, including long-acting medications (e.g., injected, implanted), over-the-counter medications, herbal products, or nutraceuticals (see Statements 3 and 4)
- Obtaining laboratory, imaging, or other evaluations to identify unrecognized contributors to the patient's delirium (e.g., infection, cardiorespiratory disease, thromboembolism, abdominal processes, head injury, medication-related toxicity, substance use; see Statement 3)
- Assessing for hypoxia or hypercapnia and providing supplemental oxygen, continuous positive airway pressure (CPAP), or ventilatory support as needed
- Ensuring pulmonary care (e.g., to avoid atelectasis)
- Correcting abnormalities in blood pressure, severe anemia, electrolytes, glucose, fluid, and acid-base status, insofar as possible
- Assessing for medical contributors to pain or distressing somatic symptoms, including postoperative pain, decubitus ulcers, degenerative joint disease, dyspnea, nausea, constipation, urinary retention, dehydration, dry mouth, and fever
- Conducting regular assessments for potential complications of delirium, including injury due to falls, pressure sores, dehydration, malnourishment, infection, venous thromboembolism, and, if applicable, postoperative or immobility-related complications
- Identifying and addressing side effects of medications, such as akathisia related to antipsychotic medications
- Identifying and addressing withdrawal symptoms related to recent use of substances (e.g., nicotine, marijuana, alcohol, sedative-hypnotics, opioids)
- Identifying and, insofar as possible, addressing co-occurring psychiatric disorders

Psychosocial support and engagement

- Assessing mental status on an ongoing basis for persistence or resolution of delirium, including a plan for follow-up assessment if delirium persists at discharge
- Providing easily readable aids to orientation and reorientation (e.g., clock, whiteboard with date)
- Ensuring availability and adequacy of dentures, glasses, hearing aids, or assistive devices
- Optimizing communication through the use of communication technologies, if indicated, and ensuring availability and use of translation services for patients whose primary language is other than English
- Providing appropriate levels of social interaction, including increasing family engagement
- Identifying and addressing distressing somatic symptoms, including pain

Table 5 Factors to consider in developing a person-centered treatment plan (*continued*)

Identifying and addressing psychological contributors to distress (e.g., fear, anxiety, boredom, over- or understimulation, co-occurring psychiatric conditions, responses to caregiver dynamics, frustration with hospital requirements and constraints)
Providing education about delirium to patients, insofar as possible, and to family members and others in the patient's support network
Personal care and environmental interventions
Ensuring early mobility
Scheduling and aiding with toileting, if necessary
Providing adequate hydration and assistance with meals, if necessary
Reviewing lines, tubes, monitoring cables, restraints, and other "tethers" and removing those that are not needed
Minimizing devices with audible alarms that can produce "alarm fatigue" in patients and in staff
Minimizing disruptions to the sleep-wake cycle (e.g., ensuring adequate daytime lighting, providing earplugs or eye masks, and minimizing as much as possible nighttime medication doses, blood draws, vital sign measurements, and the number of continuous infusions with associated intravenous pump alarms)
Providing an increased level of supervision and support, if necessary
Preventing potential complications, such as falls, pressure sores, dehydration, malnourishment, infection, venous thromboembolism, and, if applicable, postoperative or immobility-related complications
Considering personal and environmental factors that could be contributing to patient discomfort or distress (e.g., hunger/thirst, feeling hot/cold, uneven mattress or bedclothes, foreign objects left in bed, need for repositioning)

Multicomponent nonpharmacological treatments (as discussed in Statement 7) are the primary approaches used for preventing delirium (Ely 2017; Inouye 2021; Inouye et al. 2000; Marra et al. 2017; Mart et al. 2021; Oh and Park 2019; Society of Critical Care Medicine 2023). Selection of other treatment plan elements will depend in large part on the setting of care, whether delirium is present, and the patient's presenting symptoms, predisposing and precipitating risk factors, and co-occurring disorders (Maldonado 2017; Marcantonio 2017; Mattison 2020; Wilson et al. 2020). For instance, delirium that is medication induced suggests a need for medication titration or discontinuation. In patients with vision or auditory deficits, delirium symptoms may improve with the use of eyeglasses or hearing aids. Patients who are in physical restraints or who have been immobile will likely need a mobility protocol or physical rehabilitation included in their treatment plan. Patients with a history of substance use will need monitoring for signs of withdrawal and any indicated treatment. Patients with a co-occurring psychotic disorder will need standing treatment with an antipsychotic, whereas those with catatonic signs generally will be given benzodiazepines or electroconvulsive therapy (ECT) with avoidance of antipsychotic medication. Patients with pain may not always be able to ask for as-needed (i.e., prn) medications; on the other hand, they may experience side effects from frequent standing doses of pain medication such as opioids. For all patients, attention will also be needed to identify and address physical and psychological contributors to discomfort or distress (Boehm et al. 2021; Williams et al. 2020).

Person-centered treatment planning should consider how family and caregivers can be incorporated into care, as appropriate (Duong et al. 2024; Kukreja et al. 2015; Lee-Steere et al. 2024). Because of their proximity to and knowledge of the patient, family and caregivers may have an awareness of the patient's baseline level of cognition and functioning and may notice subtle changes in thinking and behavior that could inform treatment selection. For many patients with delirium, family and caregivers also play a valuable role in providing patients with support, functional assistance, and reassurance (Assa et al. 2021; Duong et al. 2024; Lange et al. 2022; McKenzie and Joy 2020; Pandhal and Van Der Wardt 2022). Facilities with restrictive visiting hour policies should consider having provisions for extended hours to allow greater family support of patients with delirium (Wu et al. 2022). In addition, for patients without involved family or for those in long-term-care settings, trained volunteers or peer specialists may be able to provide support or reassurance.

Nonpharmacological Interventions

Statement 7 – Multicomponent Nonpharmacological Interventions

APA *recommends* **(1B)** that patients with delirium or who are at risk for delirium receive multicomponent nonpharmacological interventions to manage and prevent delirium.

Implementation

Nonpharmacological interventions are an essential element in the prevention of delirium and are typically delivered as a bundle of multiple components (see Appendix C, Statement 7). Evidence is less compelling for the effects of nonpharmacological interventions on the management of delirium, but they are typically considered good clinical practice and unlikely to be harmful. Individual studies and guidelines have emphasized different combinations of nonpharmacological interventions (Table 6). Bundles of nonpharmacological interventions that have been studied most widely include the ABCDEF bundle and the Hospital Elder Life Program, but different combinations of nonpharmacological interventions also have been studied in randomized controlled trials (RCTs) (see Appendix C, Statement 7; T.J. Chen et al. 2022; Matsuura et al. 2023; Sosnowski et al. 2023). Because of their common use and the challenges of doing blinded studies with many of these interventions, it is difficult to compare the effects of these nonpharmacological bundles or to distinguish the unique effects of their individual components. Furthermore, some interventions may be implemented in different ways in various organizations. Given this, it is worth noting that studies tend to show greater benefits, particularly in preventing delirium, when a greater number of nonpharmacological interventions are used consistently (Balas et al. 2022; Barnes-Daly et al. 2017; Hshieh et al. 2018; Inouye et al. 2003; Mion et al. 2023; Pun et al. 2019).

The ABCDEF bundle includes six specific elements (Marra et al. 2017; Society of Critical Care Medicine 2023): A) **A**ssess, prevent, and manage pain; B) **B**oth spontaneous awakening trials and spontaneous breathing trials; C) **C**hoice of analgesia and sedation; D) **D**elirium: assess, prevent, and manage; E) **E**arly mobility and exercise; and F) **F**amily engagement and empowerment. Pain assessment includes obtaining information from patient self-reports but also can incorporate observed signs of pain (e.g., facial expressions, muscle tension, restlessness, vocalizations). In addition to treating pain when it is present, it is important to address pain proactively before painful procedures. Although details of the pharmacological management of pain are beyond the scope of this guideline, the advantages and disadvantages of specific medications, including their potential to worsen delirium, should be kept in mind. Nonpharmacological approaches to pain or discomfort (e.g., repositioning, application of heat or cold) also can be helpful and are often overlooked. Spontaneous awakening trials include stopping sedatives and, if possible, opioids and are accompanied by trials of spontaneous breathing in ventilated patients. In choosing sedative and analgesic medications, dexmedetomidine may be preferable to other agents (see Statements 11 and 12), and benzodiazepines should be avoided when possible (see Statement 10). Another key element of the ABCDEF bundle is the assessment of delirium using a standardized approach (see Statement

Table 6 Examples of multicomponent nonpharmacological interventions

Core component	ABCDEF bundle	Hospital Elder Life Program	Scottish Intercollegiate Guidelines Network	U.K. NICE guideline
Assessment, prevention, and management of delirium	X		X	X
Assessment, prevention, and management of pain	X		X	X
Early mobilization	X	X	X	X
Daily removal of sedation and ventilation in ICU	X			
Review medications and optimize medication choice	X		X	X
Vision protocol		X	X	
Hearing protocol		X	X	X
Oral volume repletion/ feeding assistance		X	X	X
Sleep enhancement		X	X	X
Daily visitor/orientation		X	X	X
Therapeutic activities		X		X
Family engagement	X		X	X

Note. ICU=intensive care unit; NICE=National Institute for Health and Care Excellence.

1) and the interventions to address delirium that is identified, as discussed throughout this guideline. Early mobility is important as an element of the ABCDEF bundle but also in reducing complications of prolonged immobilization such as muscle weakness and declines in functional status. If ambulation is not possible, active range of motion activities three times daily can be performed instead. Minimizing catheters, monitoring leads, restraints, and other "tethers" can also help foster greater mobility. Family engagement and empowerment are also integral to the ABCDEF bundle and can incorporate family presence on rounds, shared decision-making, and education about delirium and aspects of medical events and procedures.

The Hospital Elder Life Program interventions include a geriatric nursing assessment and interventions to address cognitive and functional impairment, dehydration, nutrition, psychoactive medication use, and discharge planning (Hshieh et al. 2018; Inouye 2021; Inouye et al. 2000). These components may include early mobilization, use of an orientation board (with date, activities, and names of team members), cognitively stimulating activities (e.g., discussion of current events, structured reminiscence, word games), interventions to enhance sleep (e.g., quiet hallways, calming music, relaxation apps, reduction in alarms, rescheduling of medications and procedures to minimize sleep disruptions), vision and hearing protocols (e.g., impacted earwax removal as needed), and appropriate use of visual and hearing aids and other adaptive equipment (e.g., magnifying lenses, large illuminated telephone keypads, large-print books, fluorescent tape on call bell). Other program elements include twice-weekly interdisciplinary rounds to discuss each patient, set goals, review issues, and track interventions, with additional interdisciplinary consultation as needed. Geriatric consultation can also be obtained with input from program staff.

A health care professional education program is provided as part of the Hospital Elder Life Program that includes formal didactic sessions, one-on-one interactions, and resource materials to educate members of the treatment team about the program elements (Hshieh et al. 2018). Linkages and communication with community agencies are used to optimize patients' transitions to home. A telephone follow-up within 7 days after discharge is also provided for all patients (Hshieh et al. 2018).

Importantly, the implementation of multicomponent nonpharmacological interventions, such as the ABCDEF bundle or Hospital Elder Life Program, is often erratic, without concerted and consistent efforts on a unit or organizational level to ensure that each intervention is completed with fidelity for each patient (Brown et al. 2022; Hshieh et al. 2018; Inouye et al. 2003; Pun et al. 2019). Nursing staff deliver or ensure the delivery of most of these interventions, and adequate nursing staffing is crucial to robust implementation. Other key features for successful implementation of multicomponent nonpharmacological interventions include gaining the support of staff and organizational leadership (including nursing and physician leaders), ensuring intervention fidelity within organizational workflows, integrating components with existing programs (e.g., geriatric care), identifying approaches to help ensure the delivery of interventions (e.g., rounding checklists, training sessions or web-based materials to educate staff or family, community volunteers to assist with some tasks, quality improvement collaboratives), using data to assess program outcomes and demonstrate benefits (e.g., decreases in delirium, fall reduction, enhanced patient and family satisfaction), changing organizational culture related to delirium assessment and interventions, and addressing program sustainability (Balas et al. 2022; Bradley et al. 2004, 2006; Brockman et al. 2023; Hshieh et al. 2018; Inouye et al. 2003; King et al. 2023; Mion et al. 2023; SteelFisher et al. 2011, 2013).

Pharmacological Interventions

Statement 8 – Principles of Medication Use

APA *recommends* **(1C)** that medications, including antipsychotic agents, be used to address neuropsychiatric disturbances of delirium only when all of the following criteria are met:

- Verbal and nonverbal de-escalation strategies have been ineffective;
- Contributing factors have been assessed and, as far as possible, addressed; and
- The disturbances cause the patient significant distress and/or present a risk of physical harm to the patient or others.

Implementation

As with any decision related to medication use, initiating a new medication in a patient with delirium requires consideration of the potential benefits of the medication as compared with the potential risks of use. Under some circumstances, neuropsychiatric disturbances of delirium might be addressed by correcting underlying contributors to delirium (see Statement 3) or by using nonpharmacological approaches such as redirection, reassurance, verbal de-escalation techniques, or family education and engagement. In other circumstances, however, nonpharmacological approaches may not be effective. Furthermore, it may not be possible to identify or resolve underlying contributors to delirium, either in a timely fashion or at all.

Delirium may be associated with a wide range of neuropsychiatric disturbances—from apathy to agitation and including psychosis, catatonia, and other neuropsychiatric manifestations. When an individual with delirium is experiencing severe and distressing neuropsychiatric disturbances, such as hallucinations, delusions, or agitation, these can require rapid intervention. This is particularly true when neuropsychiatric disturbances are serious enough to present a risk of physical harm to the patient or others. Evidence from RCTs does not support benefits of medications such as antipsychotics or benzodiazepines in the treatment of delirium (see Appendix C, Statements 9 and 10). Although data from clinical trials are limited, expert consensus based on substantial clinical experience suggests that medication, if used judiciously, can be appropriate and helpful in calming a patient with significant neuropsychiatric disturbance (Jaworska et al. 2022; see Statement 5). In addition, it may help in avoiding the use of physical restraint or reducing the duration of time in restraint. Nevertheless, if medication is being considered, it is important to be aware of biases, including racial/ethnic biases, that can influence decision-making regarding neuropsychiatric disturbances of delirium (see Statement 5). Furthermore, the duration of medication treatment should be kept as brief as possible.

Any possible benefit of medications in reducing distress or agitation must be weighed against the potential harms of medication. In individuals with neuropsychiatric disturbances of dementia, treatment with antipsychotic medications for 6–12 weeks in clinical trials has been associated with dose-dependent increases in the relative risks for mortality and other adverse effects (Maust et al. 2015; Schneider-Thoma et al. 2018; U.S. Food and Drug Administration 2005, 2008; Yunusa et al. 2019). In addition, one retrospective study showed an association between antipsychotic use and death or nonfatal cardiopulmonary arrest during hospitalization (Basciotta et al. 2020). This association was present for any type of antipsychotic medication in patients age 65 and older as well as for first-generation antipsychotic use in the full cohort of hospitalized patients and in patients with delirium (Basciotta et al. 2020). However, in RCTs of antipsychotic treatment of delirium, brief treatment with an antipsychotic such as haloperidol was not associated with significant increases in mortality or other adverse effects (Andersen-Ranberg et al. 2022, 2023a, 2023b). In addition, antipsychotic medication does not appear to increase the risk of delirium (Reisinger et al. 2023). Individuals with Parkinson's disease or Lewy body dementia are likely to be particularly sensitive to the side effects of antipsychotic medications (Devanand et al. 2024).

Other possible side effects of antipsychotic medications vary with the specific agent and are typically dose dependent (American Psychiatric Association 2021; Table 7). With short-term use of an antipsychotic to address neuropsychiatric disturbances of delirium, specific side effects include sedation, anticholinergic effects, and orthostatic hypotension. Some antipsychotic medications may also reduce the seizure threshold (Alper et al. 2007; Wu et al. 2016). Other side effects of antipsychotic medications include akathisia, which may be mistaken for agitation; dystonic reactions, which can rarely be associated with laryngospasm; and parkinsonism, with associated tremor, akinesia, and motor rigidity. Dyskinesia is typically considered to result from long-term treatment with an antipsychotic (i.e., tardive dyskinesia), but some patients develop dyskinesias with relatively short periods of treatment. In addition, patients may inadvertently be continued on an antipsychotic medication for longer periods (e.g., after discharge from the hospital), resulting in a risk for tardive dyskinesia or other tardive motor syndromes. Oropharyngeal dysphagia also has been reported with antipsychotic medication use (Miarons and Rofes 2019), which may lead to an increase in the risk of aspiration pneumonia (Herzig et al. 2017).

NMS occurs rarely but may be life-threatening because of the combination of rigidity (with elevations in serum creatine kinase levels), hyperthermia (>100.4°F/38.0°C on at least two occasions, measured orally), and sympathetic nervous system lability, including hypertension and tachycardia. Other diagnoses that may have a similar clinical presentation include malignant catatonia; malignant hyperthermia (in association with anesthetic administration); heatstroke; serotonin syndrome (in patients also taking serotonergic medications such as selective serotonin reuptake inhibitors); withdrawal from alcohol or sedative, hypnotic, or anxiolytic medications; anticholinergic syndrome; hyperthermia associated with use of stimulants and hallucinogens; central nervous system infections; limbic encephalitis; and inflammatory or autoimmune conditions (American Psychiatric Association 2022; Caroff et al. 2021; Strawn et al. 2007). If signs of apparent NMS

TABLE 7 Antipsychotic medications that may be used in the treatment of severe neuropsychiatric disturbances of delirium

	Aripiprazole	Haloperidol	Olanzapine	Quetiapine	Risperidone	Ziprasidone
Pharmacological properties[a]						
Route	Oral (tablet, disintegrating tablet,[b] solution)	Oral (tablet, concentrate), parenteral (short-acting lactate IM or IV injection)[c]	Oral (tablet, disintegrating tablet[b]), parenteral (short-acting solution for IM injection)[d]	Oral (immediate-release tablet, extended-release tablet)	Oral (tablet, disintegrating tablet,[b] solution)	Oral (capsule), parenteral (short-acting solution for IM injection)
Usual adult starting dose in delirium[e]	2 mg oral	0.5–2 mg oral/IM/IV	2.5 mg oral/IM	12.5–25 mg immediate-release oral[f]	0.25–0.5 mg oral	20 mg oral; 10–20 mg IM
Typical maximum daily dose in delirium	5–10 mg oral	20 mg oral/IM/IV	5–10 mg oral; 20–30 mg IM	100–200 mg immediate-release oral[f]	1–2 mg oral	40–80 mg oral; 20–40 mg IM
Oral bioavailability (%)	87	86	57	100	70	60 (with food)
Time to peak level[g]	3–5 hours oral	2–6 hours oral; 20 minutes IM; 2–10 minutes IV	6 hours oral; 15–45 minutes IM	1.5 hours immediate-release oral; 6 hours extended-release oral	1 hour oral	6–8 hours oral; 15–60 minutes IM
Protein binding (%)	>99	89–93	93	83	90	>99
Metabolic enzymes/transporters	CYP2D6 (major), CYP3A4 (major) substrate	CYP2D6 (major), CYP3A4 (major), CYP1A2 (minor) substrate; 50%–60% glucuronidation	CYP1A2 (major), CYP2D6 (minor) substrate; metabolized via direct glucuronidation	CYP3A4 (major), CYP2D6 (minor) substrate	CYP2D6 (major), CYP3A4 (minor) substrate; CYP2D6 weak inhibitor; ABCB1 substrate/*N*-dealkylation (minor)	CYP1A2 (minor), CYP3A4 (minor) substrate; 50-glutathione, aldehyde oxidase
Elimination half-life (adults)	75 hours, 94 hours for active metabolite, 146 hours in poor CYP2D6 metabolizers	14–37 hours	30 hours oral/IM; 1.5 times greater in older adults	6–7 hours, 12 hours for active metabolite	3–20 hours, 21–30 hours for active metabolite	7 hours oral, 2–5 hours IM

TABLE 7 Antipsychotic medications that may be used in the treatment of severe neuropsychiatric disturbances of delirium (*continued*)

	Aripiprazole	Haloperidol	Olanzapine	Quetiapine	Risperidone	Ziprasidone
Excretion	55% fecal, 25% renal	15% fecal, 30% renal (1% as unchanged medication)	30% fecal, 57% renal (7% as unchanged medication)	20% fecal, 73% renal	14% fecal, 70% renal	66% fecal, 20% renal
Renal dosing adjustments	No dosing adjustments needed; unlikely to be removed by dialysis	No dosing adjustments needed; unlikely to be removed by dialysis	No dosing adjustments needed; unlikely to be removed by dialysis	No dosing adjustments needed; unlikely to be removed by dialysis	Use lower initial dose and increase in dose increments of no more than 0.5 mg twice a day, with increases to dosages >1.5 mg twice a day occurring at intervals of at least 1 week if CrCl is <30 mL/minute; not significantly dialyzed	IM formulation should be used with caution because it includes a cyclodextrin excipient, which is cleared by the kidney; unlikely to be removed by dialysis
Hepatic dosing adjustments	No dosing adjustments needed	No dosing adjustments provided	No dosing adjustments provided (except in combination with fluoxetine), but use with caution because of reports of hepatitis and liver injury	Use initial dose of 25 mg immediate release and increase by no more than 25–50 mg immediate-release daily in the presence of hepatic impairment	Use lower initial dose with mild to severe hepatic impairment (Child-Pugh class A, B, or C) and slower titration rate with severe hepatic impairment (Child-Pugh class C); increase in dose increments of no more than 0.5 mg twice a day, with increases to dosages >1.5 mg twice a day occurring at intervals of at least 1 week	No dosing adjustments provided, but use with caution because of extensive hepatic metabolism

TABLE 7 Antipsychotic medications that may be used in the treatment of severe neuropsychiatric disturbances of delirium (*continued*)

	Aripiprazole	Haloperidol	Olanzapine	Quetiapine	Risperidone	Ziprasidone
Relative frequency of side effects[h]						
Akathisia	++	+++	++	+	++	++
Parkinsonism	+	+++	++	+	++	+
Dystonia	+	+++	+	+	++	+
Tardive dyskinesia	+	+++	+	+	++	+
Hyperprolactinemia	+	+++	++	+	+++	++
Anticholinergic	+	+	++	++	+	+
Sedation	+	+	+++	+++	++	++
Seizures	+	+	++	++	+	+
Orthostasis	+	+	++	++	++	++
QT prolongation	+	++	++	++	++	+++
Weight gain	+	++	+++	++	++	+
Hyperlipidemia	+	+	+++	+++	+	+
Glucose abnormalities	+	+	+++	++	++	+
Comments[i,j,k,l]	Reduce dose in poor CYP2D6 metabolizers or with concomitant CYP3A4 or CYP2D6 inhibitors. Check FDA safety alert for impulse-control disorders (e.g., gambling, binge eating).		Administer IM slowly, deep into muscle; do not give subcutaneously. Concomitant use of IM olanzapine and IM or IV benzodiazepine (e.g., within 1 hour) is not recommended because of potential for excessive sedation or cardiorespiratory depression. Women may need a lower dose. 40% of oral doses are removed via first-pass metabolism.	Reduce to one-sixth of the original dose after starting a strong CYP3A4 inhibitor. Strong CYP3A4 inducers may decrease serum concentration of quetiapine, and as much as a 5-fold increase in dose may be needed to maintain therapeutic benefit. If the CYP3A4 inducer is stopped, dose reduction is needed within 7–14 days of inducer discontinuation.	Reduce dose with concomitant strong CYP2D6 inhibitor. Strong CYP3A4 inhibitors may increase serum risperidone concentration, requiring a dosage reduction. Strong CYP3A4 inducers may decrease serum concentration of risperidone and metabolite, requiring a dosage increase. Inform patients with phenylketonuria that oral disintegrating tablets contain phenylalanine. Check labeling for compatibility of oral solution with other liquids. Intraoperative floppy iris syndrome reported.	Give capsules with at least 500 calories of food. See labeling for reconstitution and storage of IM solution.

TABLE 7 Antipsychotic medications that may be used in the treatment of severe neuropsychiatric disturbances of delirium (*continued*)

Note. This table includes information compiled from multiple sources. Detailed information on issues such as dose regimen, dose adjustments, medication administration procedures, handling precautions, and storage can be found in product labeling. We recommend that readers consult product labeling information for authoritative information on these medications.

Droperidol is a first-generation antipsychotic medication that is available in a parenteral formulation. It has been used for the prevention and treatment of postoperative nausea and vomiting and also has efficacy in treating agitation. Droperidol has an FDA boxed warning recommending that it be used only when there has not been an acceptable response to other adequate treatments. The boxed warning also recommends that a 12-lead electrocardiogram (ECG) be done before administration to assess for QTc interval prolongation and that ECG monitoring be done during treatment and for 2–3 hours after completing treatment to monitor for QTc interval prolongation and serious arrhythmias (e.g., torsades de pointes). For these reasons, droperidol is rarely used in patients with delirium.

Chlorpromazine is a first-generation antipsychotic medication, available as an oral tablet, oral concentrate, and parenteral formulation. It has occasionally been used intravenously in patients with delirium whose agitation has not been able to be addressed with other medications and who cannot take oral medications, such as in palliative settings. When used, it is generally administered intravenously in low doses (e.g., initially 10–25 mg/day total) and titrated to clinical effect. Sedation and reductions in blood pressure are relatively common side effects, and extrapyramidal side effects and ECG changes also may be observed.

Brexpiprazole is a second-generation antipsychotic medication, available as an oral tablet, that is infrequently used in patients with delirium. It has a long half-life and may require dose adjustment in patients with renal impairment, moderate or severe hepatic impairment, poor metabolism through CYP2D6, or concomitant use of moderate/strong CYP2D6 or CYP3A4 inhibitors.

Patients with Parkinson's disease or dementia with Lewy bodies have an increased sensitivity to medication-induced parkinsonism, and a second-generation antipsychotic medication, such as quetiapine, is preferable to medications such as haloperidol or risperidone.

CrCl=creatinine clearance; CYP=cytochrome P450; FDA=U.S. Food and Drug Administration; IM=intramuscular; IV=intravenous.

[a]Pharmacological properties may differ with patient age (particularly in older individuals), body size and composition, organ system impairment, and other factors.

[b]The oral disintegrating tablet formulation is absorbed enterally and not sublingually. Thus, its absorption and other pharmacokinetic properties are similar to those of other oral formulations. Oral disintegrating tablets should not be split or crushed.

[c]Haloperidol is available in a long-acting intramuscular decanoate formulation and a short-acting parenteral formulation. Only the short-acting parenteral formulation is appropriate for use in patients with delirium unless a patient is already taking the long-acting injectable decanoate formulation for a preexisting psychotic disorder.

[d]The parenteral formulation of olanzapine has also been used intravenously (typical dose=2.5–5 mg) and most often in emergency and critical care settings for the treatment of agitation.

[e]Suggested starting doses are based on expert consensus. Typically, the starting dose in a patient with delirium is one-half, or less, of the recommended starting dose for the same medication in adults with other psychiatric conditions.

[f]Although an extended-release formulation of quetiapine is available, the immediate-release formulation is suggested for use in individuals with delirium.

[g]The initial onset of action of a medication may precede the time at which the peak medication level is reached.

[h]The relative frequency of side effects is designated by +=seldom; ++=sometimes; +++=often.

[i]Patients with dementia-related psychosis treated with antipsychotics are at an increased risk of death compared with placebo, and an FDA boxed warning applies to all antipsychotic medications. Antipsychotic agents with an indication for augmentation treatment in major depressive disorder or bipolar depression (e.g., aripiprazole, olanzapine, quetiapine) have an additional black box warning related to increased risk of suicidal thinking/behaviors in children, adolescents, and young adults taking antidepressants.

[j]Administration can occur without regard to food or other medications unless specifically noted.

[k]Tablets can be crushed or split unless specifically noted.

[l]As described by Pugh et al. (1973), Child-Pugh class A corresponds to a Child-Pugh score of 5–6, class B corresponds to a Child-Pugh score of 7–9, and class C corresponds to a Child-Pugh score of 10–15.

Package insert references. Abilify 2022; Aripiprazole orally disintegrating tablets 2018; Aripiprazole solution 2016; Chlorpromazine hydrochloride concentrate 2023; Chlorpromazine hydrochloride injection 2023; Chlorpromazine hydrochloride tablets 2024; Geodon 2022; Haloperidol 2008, 2019; Haloperidol lactate 2008; Haldol lactate injection 2020; Haloperidol lactate injection 2011; Haloperidol lactate oral solution 2016; Haloperidol lactate oral solution USP 2020; Haloperidol tablets 2015, 2019; Risperdal 2020, 2022; Risperidone orally disintegrating tablets 2019; Seroquel 2022; Seroquel XR 2022; Zyprexa 2021.

Source. American Psychiatric Association 2021; Curry et al. 2023; Hasuo et al. 2018; Hospira 2021; Hui et al. 2020; Hunt et al. 2021; Lexi-Drugs 2024; Martel et al. 2016; Micromedex 2024; Procyshyn et al. 2023; Roppolo et al. 2020; Thom et al. 2019; Tsai et al. 2021; Wang et al. 2022; Wilson et al. 2012.

develop, antipsychotic medications should be discontinued and supportive treatment should be provided to maintain hydration, treat fever, and address cardiovascular, renal, or other abnormalities (Caroff et al. 2021; Guinart et al. 2021; Strawn et al. 2007). Assistance with emergency management of NMS is recommended and can be obtained through NMSContact (https://my.mhaus.org/page/contactmhaus).

Treatment with an antipsychotic medication may be associated with QTc interval prolongation and, if significant, an increased risk for torsades de pointes, which may lead to life-threatening consequences (e.g., ventricular fibrillation, sudden death) (Funk et al. 2018). A QTc interval greater than 500 msec is sometimes viewed as a threshold for concern; however, "there is no absolute QTc interval at which a psychotropic should not be used" (Funk et al. 2018, p. 2). In addition, with marked tachycardia or bradycardia (i.e., significantly greater than or less than, respectively, 60 beats/minute), alternative formulas may need to be used because the QTc interval will, respectively, be overestimated or underestimated by the formula used to calculate QTc intervals in automated electrocardiogram (ECG) reports. Among antipsychotic medications that are available in parenteral formulations, chlorpromazine, droperidol, and ziprasidone appear to be associated with the greatest risk of QTc interval prolongation (Funk et al. 2018). Concern has also been raised about QTc interval prolongation with haloperidol, and the U.S. Food and Drug Administration (FDA) recommends cardiac monitoring of patients when intravenous haloperidol is used (Meyer-Massetti et al. 2010). Despite this, the risk of significant QTc interval changes appears to be relatively small, particularly in the doses studied in clinical trials of patients with delirium (Beach et al. 2020). For example, in a large RCT of haloperidol (n=192) as compared with ziprasidone (n=190) or placebo (n=184), QTc interval prolongation that resulted in the holding of medication was more common in the ziprasidone group (2% of doses) than in the haloperidol group or placebo group (1% of doses in each group) (Stollings et al. 2024). In another large multicenter placebo-controlled randomized trial of intravenous haloperidol (N=987; 2.5 mg three times daily plus 2.5 mg as needed up to a total maximum daily dose of 20 mg) in adult ICU patients, QTc interval prolongation was associated with medication discontinuation in 2.4% of the haloperidol group as compared with 1.4% of the placebo group (Andersen-Ranberg et al. 2022). Many other antipsychotic agents also have FDA warnings or possible risks for QTc interval prolongation (Funk et al. 2018). Additional factors that influence the risk of QTc interval prolongation include whether the patient is taking other medications that are known to prolong QTc intervals; whether the patient has factors that would influence medication metabolism, leading to higher blood levels of a medication (e.g., poor metabolizer status, pharmacokinetic drug-drug interactions, hepatic or renal disease, medication toxicity); whether the patient is known to have a significant cardiac risk factor (e.g., congenital long QT syndrome, structural or functional cardiac disease, bradycardia, family history of sudden cardiac death); or other factors associated with an increased risk of torsades de pointes (e.g., female sex; advanced age; personal history of medication-induced QTc interval prolongation; severe acute illness; starvation; risk or presence of hypokalemia, hypomagnesemia, or hypocalcemia) (Funk et al. 2018).

If the clinician decides to begin an antipsychotic to reduce neuropsychiatric disturbances of delirium, antipsychotic medications are usually begun on an as-needed (i.e., prn) basis and should be started at a low dose, typically half or less than that of a usual adult starting dose (Table 7). Although medications are often given in combination when treating agitation (e.g., haloperidol plus lorazepam, haloperidol plus diphenhydramine), using an antipsychotic medication alone is preferred in a patient with delirium and in older individuals because of a potential increase in sedation, added anticholinergic effects, and worsening of delirium (Korczak et al. 2016; Yap et al. 2019). Before administering additional doses of antipsychotic or other sedating medications, the clinician should allow a sufficient period for the initial medication to take effect. This is dependent on the route of administration and the pharmacological properties of the medication but may require 5–15 minutes for intravenous doses and 30–45 minutes for intramuscular or oral doses

(Table 7). If an additional dose of a medication appears to be needed after waiting an appropriate time for it to take effect, a second dose should be the same or lower than the initial dose because of the cumulative nature of a repeat dose. Alternatively, a different medication could be tried instead of repeating the dose of the initial medication. Inclusion of a maximal daily dose as part of the medication order can help avoid excess sedation or other side effects of treatment. In addition, orders for antipsychotic medication should be limited in duration (e.g., 3–5 days), and potential benefits and risks of use should be reviewed before continuing treatment. Before discharge, the need for continued treatment should be reassessed (see Statement 15).

Statement 9 – Antipsychotic Agents

APA *recommends* **(1C)** that antipsychotic agents not be used to prevent delirium or hasten its resolution.

Implementation

Evidence from RCTs does not support benefits of antipsychotic medications in preventing or treating delirium (see Appendix C, Statement 9). Because of the potential risks associated with antipsychotic medication treatment and the lack of apparent benefits in preventing or treating delirium, the use of an antipsychotic for these purposes is not recommended.

An antipsychotic medication sometimes may be appropriate when an individual with delirium is experiencing severe neuropsychiatric disturbances that cause the patient significant distress and/or present a risk of physical harm to the patient or others (see Statement 8). However, such use of antipsychotic medication should be time-limited (e.g., at most 3–5 days per order), with frequent review of the need for further use. An antipsychotic medication also can be initiated or continued in a patient with delirium superimposed on a co-occurring psychotic disorder (American Psychiatric Association 2021). If a patient has been receiving treatment with an antipsychotic medication to address severe neuropsychiatric disturbances related to dementia, the rationale and history of use should be reviewed to determine whether the patient would potentially benefit from an attempt to taper the antipsychotic medication (American Psychiatric Association 2016).

Statement 10 – Benzodiazepines

APA *recommends* **(1C)** that benzodiazepines not be used in patients with delirium or who are at risk for delirium, including those with preexisting cognitive impairment, unless there is a specific indication for their use.

Implementation

In patients with delirium or who are at risk for delirium, the use of benzodiazepines is not typically recommended (Curry et al. 2023; Shenvi et al. 2020). Randomized studies of midazolam or lorazepam in the treatment or prevention of delirium are limited in number but have not shown benefits of benzodiazepine treatment as compared with other treatment options (see Appendix C, Statement 10). Although perioperative use of a benzodiazepine does not appear to increase the likelihood of delirium overall (Wang et al. 2023), the incidence and duration of delirium appear to be greater with the use of midazolam than with dexmedetomidine (Hassan et al. 2021; He et al. 2018; Maldonado et al. 2009; Yu et al. 2017). Furthermore, in ICU patients, the duration of mechanical ventilation is somewhat greater with midazolam than with dexmedetomidine (Jakob et al. 2012), whereas no differences have been noted on most other outcomes. In observational and database studies in other settings, some research suggests that delirium may be increased by the use of a benzodiazepine, but evidence is mixed, and its reliability is low (Reisinger et al. 2023; see also Appendix C, Statement 10).

Side effects of benzodiazepines may add to the potential risks of treatment, particularly in older individuals and those with preexisting cognitive impairment (American Geriatrics Society Beers Criteria® Update Expert Panel 2023; Shenvi et al. 2020). Such effects may include an increased risk of falls, oversedation, or respiratory depression (American Geriatrics Society Beers Criteria® Update Expert Panel 2023; Engstrom et al. 2023; Korczak et al. 2016; Roppolo et al. 2020; Shenvi et al. 2020; Wilson et al. 2012; Yap et al. 2019). Paradoxical increases in agitation also have been reported with benzodiazepines but appear to be uncommon (Champion et al. 2021; Gonzalez et al. 2023; Mancuso et al. 2004).

With these caveats, it is important to note that in some circumstances, treatment with a benzodiazepine still may be indicated in a patient with delirium or at risk for delirium (Table 8).

TABLE 8 **Factors suggesting that a benzodiazepine may be indicated in a patient with delirium**
High likelihood of alcohol or sedative-hypnotic withdrawal by clinical history and symptoms
Acute intoxication from anticholinergic agents, stimulant use, psychedelic drugs, or multiple unknown substances
Prominent signs of catatonia
Neuroleptic malignant syndrome
Serotonin syndrome
Autoimmune encephalitis
Long-standing use of a benzodiazepine before hospitalization, for which discontinuation may prompt withdrawal symptoms or symptom rebound
Seizure disorder that requires the use of a benzodiazepine for adequate seizure control

In individuals whose clinical history and symptoms suggest apparent alcohol or sedative-hypnotic withdrawal, treatment with a fixed dose of a benzodiazepine (i.e., diazepam, chlordiazepoxide, lorazepam) is effective in reducing the likelihood of alcohol withdrawal seizures (Bahji et al. 2022) and is more effective than the use of anticonvulsant medication (Lai et al. 2022). The available studies also suggest that diazepam can reduce the incidence of delirium tremens (Bahji et al. 2022). Of the benzodiazepines, lorazepam is shorter acting, is rapidly conjugated to a glucuronide in the liver, does not have active metabolites or interactions with CYP enzymes, and can be given orally, intravenously, or intramuscularly because it has good intramuscular absorption (Procyshyn et al. 2023); thus, it may be preferable to diazepam or chlordiazepoxide in older individuals in an acute care setting.

In a patient who appears to be intoxicated and is experiencing agitation in an acute care setting, a benzodiazepine is generally preferable to an antipsychotic medication if the cause of intoxication is unclear or appears related to anticholinergic agents, stimulants, or psychedelic drugs (Engstrom et al. 2023; Roppolo et al. 2020; Shenvi et al. 2020; Wilson et al. 2012). By contrast, administration of a benzodiazepine to treat agitation is not recommended in a patient who is intoxicated with alcohol or a sedative-hypnotic because of potential additive effects (Curry et al. 2023; Engstrom et al. 2023; Roppolo et al. 2020; Shenvi et al. 2020; Wilson et al. 2012).

Catatonia may co-occur with delirium, and these features may warrant treatment with a benzodiazepine (Appiani et al. 2023; Oldham and Lee 2015; Wilson et al. 2017). Other acute conditions in which the use of a benzodiazepine may be indicated include NMS, serotonin syndrome, autoimmune encephalitis, and status epilepticus (Connell et al. 2023; Denysenko et al. 2018; Huang et al. 2020; Jaimes-Albornoz et al. 2022; Moss et al. 2019; Rogers et al. 2023; van Rensburg and Decloedt 2019; Zaman et al. 2019).

On a longer-term basis, benzodiazepines may be an appropriate treatment for several conditions, such as seizure disorders, severe anxiety, panic attacks, restless legs syndrome, and rapid eye movement sleep behavior disorder. In some instances, benzodiazepine treatment for these conditions may be initiated while a patient is also experiencing delirium. More often, a patient will be treated with a benzodiazepine before the development of delirium, and questions may arise as to whether the benzodiazepine should be continued. For a patient whose condition has been stable during long-term treatment with a benzodiazepine, no immediate change will be needed. In addition, whatever the indication for long-standing benzodiazepine treatment, withdrawal symptoms or symptom rebound may occur with discontinuation. If the clinician decides to reduce or stop a benzodiazepine, the time needed to do so will depend on the duration of treatment and the total daily dose (American Society of Addiction Medicine 2025; Markota et al. 2016). Furthermore, dose reduction may need to occur even more slowly toward the end of the tapering process (American Society of Addiction Medicine 2025; Markota et al. 2016).

Statement 11 – Dexmedetomidine to Prevent Delirium

APA *suggests* **(2B)** that dexmedetomidine be used rather than other sedating agents to prevent delirium in patients who are undergoing major surgery or receiving mechanical ventilation in a critical care setting.

Implementation

Dexmedetomidine has both benefits and potential risks in patients at risk for delirium. Consequently, the decision to use dexmedetomidine varies with the individual patient's physical status and co-occurring conditions. Nevertheless, in patients at risk for delirium who are undergoing major surgery or receiving mechanical ventilation in a critical care setting, the possibility of using dexmedetomidine may be raised with the patient's critical care intensivist, surgeon, anesthesiologist, or other health care professionals on the treatment team.

In patients undergoing major surgery and in those receiving mechanical ventilation in a critical care setting, evidence shows a significant reduction in the incidence of delirium when dexmedetomidine is used (see Appendix C, Statement 11). The superiority of dexmedetomidine in terms of delirium incidence is also seen when dexmedetomidine is compared head-to-head with other sedating medications (e.g., haloperidol, propofol, midazolam, clonidine, sufentanil) (see Appendix C, Statement 11). In terms of other outcomes, the benefits of dexmedetomidine are less robust, but a shorter period of mechanical ventilation and shorter lengths of stay in the ICU and the hospital have been observed in many studies of dexmedetomidine as compared with placebo or other sedating medications (Lewis et al. 2022; see Appendix C, Statement 11). Some, but not all, studies have reported improvements in sleep parameters in patients who received nocturnal dexmedetomidine compared with placebo (Knauert et al. 2023), and improvements in sleep could indirectly affect delirium incidence.

Dexmedetomidine binds to both presynaptic and postsynaptic α_2-adrenergic receptors and is more selective for α_2-adrenergic receptors than is clonidine (Weerink et al. 2017). Central effects in the locus coeruleus are thought to account for the ability of dexmedetomidine to produce sedation without respiratory depression (Weerink et al. 2017). It may also act on α_2-adrenergic receptors in the spinal cord to modify pain sensation (Weerink et al. 2017). Other physiological effects of dexmedetomidine include bradycardia and hypotension, which are estimated to occur in 13% and 25% of patients, respectively, with serious effect in 0.9% and 1.7% of patients, respectively (Keating 2015). Because of these effects, greater caution may be needed in patients with heart block, bradycardia, severe ventricular dysfunction, chronic hypertension, or hypovolemia (Hospira 2023; Lexi-Drugs

2024; Micromedex 2024). Some patients also experience an increase rather than a decrease in blood pressure with dexmedetomidine (Keating 2015). These effects on blood pressure and heart rate appear to be mediated by peripheral effects on vascular smooth muscles and vascular endothelial cells (Weerink et al. 2017).

In addition to potential effects on cardiovascular parameters, one post hoc Bayesian analysis suggested that mortality was increased when dexmedetomidine was used in nonsurgical patients younger than 65 years who were mechanically ventilated and critically ill but was reduced in other patient subgroups (Shehabi et al. 2021). In other randomized trials, mortality outcomes in samples as a whole did not differ for dexmedetomidine as compared with placebo or another medication (see Appendix C, Statement 11). In addition, a retrospective propensity-matched analysis found no difference in mortality based on age or postoperative status (Zhao et al. 2024).

Dexmedetomidine provides light sedation, which is advantageous in terms of early patient mobilization, but needs to be used in combination with other agents or substituted with an alternative agent if deep sedation is required (Lexi-Drugs 2024). In addition, if amnesia is crucial, another agent needs to be used instead of or in addition to dexmedetomidine because dexmedetomidine does not have reliable amnestic effects (Lexi-Drugs 2024). High fever has been associated with dexmedetomidine use in several case reports and may need to be distinguished from other causes of fever, such as infection, malignant hyperthermia, or NMS (Krüger et al. 2017).

Dexmedetomidine is administered as a continuous intravenous infusion that is typically titrated to achieve the desired clinical effect (Ber et al. 2020; Hospira 2023; Keating 2015; Lexi-Drugs 2024; Micromedex 2024; Weerink et al. 2017). Although the manufacturer's labeling in the United States recommends a treatment duration of up to 24 hours (Hospira 2023; Lexi-Drugs 2024), dexmedetomidine infusions lasting up to 14 days have shown ongoing safety and efficacy (Ber et al. 2020). In terms of pharmacokinetics, dexmedetomidine is highly bound to plasma proteins and metabolized by CYP enzymes and uridine 5′-diphospho-glucuronosyltransferase (UGT) (Ber et al. 2020; Keating 2015). Because clearance of the medication occurs almost entirely through the liver, lower doses of intravenous dexmedetomidine are needed in individuals with hepatic function impairment (Weerink et al. 2017). There is substantial interindividual variability in estimates of pharmacokinetic parameters (e.g., volume of distribution) in relation to organ system function in critical illnesses (Tse et al. 2018).

When patients receive doses at the upper end of the dose range or longer-term infusions, abrupt cessation of intravenous dexmedetomidine may be associated with withdrawal symptoms, including hypertension, tachycardia, nausea, vomiting, and agitation (Hospira 2023; Lexi-Drugs 2024; Micromedex 2024). An increase in blood pressure may be more likely to occur with abrupt dexmedetomidine discontinuation in patients with preexisting hypertension. In addition, withdrawal symptoms may be more likely in patients who are simultaneously discontinued from opioids or benzodiazepines (Pathan et al. 2021). It is not clear whether weaning of dexmedetomidine affects the likelihood of withdrawal symptoms on cessation (Pathan et al. 2021), but gradual discontinuation of dexmedetomidine has been suggested as a possible strategy (Lexi-Drugs 2024). A transition to clonidine (0.1–0.3 mg orally or enterally every 6–8 hours or transdermal clonidine 100 μg/24-hour patch) also may be helpful in reducing the likelihood or magnitude of withdrawal symptoms (Glaess et al. 2020). Guanfacine (0.5–1 mg two to three times daily) has been suggested as an alternative to clonidine because of its lesser effects on the vascular system as compared with the central nervous system (Fetters et al. 2022).

Statement 12 – Dexmedetomidine in Patients With Delirium

APA *suggests* **(2C)** that when patients with delirium are sedated for mechanical ventilation in a critical care setting, dexmedetomidine be used rather than other sedating agents.

Implementation

In patients who have delirium and are sedated for mechanical ventilation in a critical care setting, the use of dexmedetomidine appears to be associated with a faster resolution of delirium and fewer days with delirium than comparison treatments (see Appendix C, Statement 12). Potential risks of dexmedetomidine also exist, as described in Statement 11. Consequently, the decision to use dexmedetomidine varies with the individual patient's physical status and co-occurring conditions and can be raised with the patient's critical care intensivist or other health care professionals on the treatment team.

Although dexmedetomidine, administered as a sublingual film, has not been studied for its sedative properties in patients with delirium, it has been found to be beneficial in the treatment of agitation in patients with schizophrenia, schizoaffective disorder, and bipolar disorder (Citrome et al. 2022; Preskorn et al. 2022).

Statement 13 – Melatonin and Ramelteon

APA *suggests* **(2C)** that melatonin and ramelteon not be used to prevent or treat delirium.

Implementation

Melatonin is an endogenous hormone that affects sleep through the regulation of circadian rhythm (Minich et al. 2022; Moon et al. 2022a, 2022b). Sleep is a problem for most hospitalized patients because of noise, ambient light, monitoring devices, tubes and intravenous lines, and interruptions of sleep for medications, vital signs, and other interventions (Showler et al. 2023). Circadian rhythms are often disrupted, and medications can affect sleep patterns and rapid eye movement sleep (Showler et al. 2023). Sleep changes are common with aging, and hospitalized patients may have had sleep difficulties prior to admission (Showler et al. 2023).

Disruption of the sleep-wake cycle is common in individuals with delirium (American Psychiatric Association 2022). Consequently, melatonin and ramelteon are sometimes prescribed with the goal of preventing or treating delirium through their effects on sleep. Although some studies have shown small benefits of exogenous melatonin and melatonin agonists, such as ramelteon, in patients with delirium or at risk for delirium, the bulk of the evidence, when taken together, shows small or no effects of these agents on preventing or treating delirium (e.g., decreasing delirium incidence, severity, or duration; reducing mortality in patients with delirium) (see Appendix C, Statement 13). For these reasons, we suggest that melatonin and ramelteon not be used to prevent or treat delirium.

Although this guideline statement is specific to delirium, in hospitalized patients, melatonin and ramelteon are often prescribed for sleep (Rinehart et al. 2024; White et al. 2023), with unclear benefits (Heavner et al. 2024; Showler et al. 2023). For treatment of acute and chronic insomnia, in general, evidence suggests that melatonin and ramelteon have few side effects, but the benefits are also limited (De Crescenzo et al. 2022; Maruani et al. 2023; Sateia et al. 2017). If melatonin or ramelteon is used, however, it is important to recognize that to achieve a physiological effect, these medications require timing of their administration to the patient's circadian phase (Moon et al. 2022a, 2022b), typically 30–120 minutes before bedtime when prescribed for insomnia (Lexi-Drugs 2024; Micromedex 2024; Minich et al. 2022). Attention to possible drug-drug interactions is also needed because melatonin and ramelteon are both metabolized via CYP1A2, CYP2C9, and CYP2C19, and ramelteon is also metabolized via CYP3A4 (Lexi-Drugs 2024; Micromedex 2024; Minich et al. 2022). With melatonin, an additional concern is the lack of standardization of doses and preparations of natural products (Erland and Saxena 2017).

Transitions of Care

Statement 14 – Medication Review at Transitions of Care

APA *recommends* **(1C)** that in patients with delirium or who are at risk for delirium, a detailed medication review, medication reconciliation, and reassessment of the indications for medications, including psychotropic medications, be conducted at transitions of care within the hospital.

Implementation

Several studies have found benefits of medication review in decreasing the incidence, severity, or duration of delirium (Burton et al. 2021a; Drewas et al. 2022; van Velthuijsen et al. 2018). In addition, medication review is often a component of multicomponent nonpharmacological interventions for patients at risk for delirium (Burton et al. 2021a; see Statement 7).

For hospitalized patients, transitions of care are common and may involve changing levels of care (e.g., critical care to step-down unit or general unit), changing services (e.g., medicine to surgery), changing units (e.g., in relation to bed availability), or changing care teams. Often, several such changes may occur at once. Consequently, transitions of care may contribute to gaps in communication, and the use of structured handoff tools has been suggested to reduce such gaps (Buljac-Samardzic et al. 2020; Müller et al. 2018; Rosenthal et al. 2018). In patients with delirium or who are at risk for delirium, a detailed medication review, medication reconciliation, and reassessment of the indications for all medications at transitions of care can ensure that medication-related plans are communicated correctly. Such a review also provides an opportunity to identify medications that may be contributing to delirium or constitute a risk for delirium, as discussed in Statements 3 and 4. Evidence suggests that the medication reconciliation process can be more efficient and more effective when done by a pharmacist, pharmacy technician, or other designated staff member who has knowledge of medications (Marshall et al. 2022; Mekonnen et al. 2016b; Schnipper et al. 2023). Table 9 provides a list of key questions related to medication review and reconciliation at transitions of care.

Documentation at transitions of care should note whether home medications have been substituted with another medication because of formulary considerations or whether home medications are on hold for another reason (e.g., lack of a parenteral formulation to use while a patient is not taking oral

TABLE 9 Medication-related considerations at transitions of care

Is the patient's current list of medications accurate?
Has medication reconciliation been completed?
Are there any medications included in clinical notes, orders, and medication administration records that differ from those on the list of reconciled medications?
Were any medications that the patient is supposed to be taking inadvertently discontinued?
Did the patient receive any long-acting injectable or implanted medications prior to hospitalization or during the hospitalization that are not listed with the other medications (e.g., antipsychotic medications, naltrexone, contraceptives, glucagon-like peptide-1 receptor agonists)?

Table 9 Medication-related considerations at transitions of care (*continued*)

Are any adjustments to the patient's medications needed?

Do any medications need to be added or prior medications resumed?

Are any of the patient's current medications likely to increase the risk or duration of delirium? If so, is adjustment of medication dose or discontinuation of the medication warranted?

Are any medication-related side effects present that would warrant adjustment of medication dose or discontinuation of the medication?

Do any of the patient's current medications interact with other medications that they are taking? If so, are adjustments in medication doses needed, or should the medication be discontinued? Should additional monitoring be instituted for side effects or to ensure that medications are producing their intended benefits?

Are any of the patient's current medications potentially problematic in terms of their current diagnoses? (e.g., renally excreted medications with acute kidney injury)

Do any medication doses need to be adjusted because of a change in renal or hepatic function?

Are there any medications, including "as-needed" (i.e., prn) medications (e.g., for reasons such as pain, nausea, agitation, sleep, gastrointestinal reflux, or constipation), that may be able to be discontinued?

Does the documentation at the transition of care include all necessary communications about the patient's medications that will be relevant to future care and decision-making?

Were any of the patient's medications initiated during the hospitalization? If so, is there a clear description of the reason that the medication was begun?

Is the patient taking a psychotropic medication either as a standing dose or as-needed (i.e., prn) medication? If so, is there a clear description of the reason that the medication has been prescribed?

Was the patient taking medications prior to admission that have been stopped? If so, is the reason for stopping those medications clear (e.g., nonformulary, oral formulation in a patient who was not able to take medications orally, adverse effects of medication, lack of therapeutic benefit)? Do any of these stopped medications need to be resumed?

Was the patient taking over-the-counter medications, herbal products, supplements, or nutraceuticals at home for which they may need instructions (i.e., to continue or stop) at discharge?

Are any of the patient's medications time-limited, with a defined stop date (e.g., antibiotics)? If so, is this information noted, including a discontinuation date?

Are there specific plans to increase or decrease the dose of specific medications or discontinue a medication prior to discharge? If so, are these described clearly?

medications). If a home medication has been discontinued with no intention to resume it, this should be communicated along with the reason for discontinuation. The rationale for changes in medication doses or addition of new medications during hospitalization is also important to document so that this will be clear to subsequent clinicians (Jaworska et al. 2022). Planned increases or decreases in medication doses also should be noted. If a medication is being given for a specified number of days (e.g., a course of antibiotics, postoperative pain medication), those treatment durations should be specified. Documentation should list a specific date on which the course of treatment is expected to end to avoid confusion caused by copying and pasting electronic record information from earlier days.

Information also should be noted on any long-acting medications (e.g., long-acting injectable formulations of antipsychotic medications, naltrexone, contraceptives, glucagon-like peptide-1 receptor agonists; implantable formulations of contraceptives), as-needed (i.e., prn) medications, and over-the-counter medications, herbal products, supplements, or nutraceuticals that may have been taken at home or during the hospital stay. Medication review, reconciliation, and reassessment are also critical to identify medications, such as antipsychotics, that are started during the hospital stay but are no longer needed. Once prescribed, these medications are often continued at transfers of care and hospital discharge, increasing the risk of adverse effects (Boncyk et al. 2021; D'Angelo et al. 2019; Dixit et al. 2021; Flurie et al. 2015; Johnson et al. 2017; Lambert et al. 2021; Markota et al. 2016). Other goals of medication review include identifying agents that may be producing side effects or contributing to drug-drug or drug-disease interactions through pharmacokinetic or pharmacodynamic effects (see Statement 4).

Statement 15 – Follow-Up Planning at Transitions of Care

APA *recommends* **(1C)** that when patients with delirium are transferred to another setting of care, plans for follow-up include:

- Continued assessments for persistence of delirium;
- Detailed medication review, medication reconciliation, and reassessment of the indications for medications, including psychotropic medications;
- Assessment of the consequences of delirium (e.g., posttraumatic symptoms, cognitive impairment); and
- Psychoeducation about delirium for patients and their care partners.

Implementation

As with transitions of care within the hospital, clear handoff communications and a detailed review and reconciliation of medications are important when a patient is transferred to another setting (see Statement 14 and Table 9). This process should include reassessment of the indications for medications, including psychotropic medications. Evidence suggests that the medication reconciliation process can be more efficient and more effective when done by a pharmacist, pharmacy technician, or other designated staff member who has knowledge of medications (Marshall et al. 2022; Mekonnen et al. 2016b; Schnipper et al. 2023).

Multiple retrospective studies suggest that a significant fraction of hospitalized individuals with delirium were administered an antipsychotic or sedative medication during the inpatient stay and continued taking it after discharge (Boncyk et al. 2021; Burry et al. 2023; Dixit et al. 2021; Flurie et al. 2015; Johnson et al. 2017; Lambert et al. 2021; Welk et al. 2021). Medication review at the time of transfer or discharge can identify medications that can be discontinued or that need to be tapered and then stopped (Adeola et al. 2018; American Geriatrics Society Beers Criteria® Update Expert Panel 2023; D'Angelo et al. 2019; Kram et al. 2019; McDonald et al. 2022; O'Mahony et al. 2015; Redmond et al. 2018; Reeve 2020; Stuart et al. 2020; Tamblyn et al. 2019; see Appendix C, Statement 14). If a medication, such as an antipsychotic medication, has been started during the hospital stay to address agitation or psychosis due to delirium, it should be stopped when those symptoms abate. Antipsychotic medications should not be continued after discharge unless prescribed for some other purpose (e.g., preexisting psychiatric condition).

Follow-up care is critical for patients who have had delirium because symptom resolution may vary widely, from hours to days to weeks, or even months in some patients (Oldham et al. 2017). Despite this, persistent delirium is often unrecognized and may reflect ongoing physical health issues that need further evaluation or treatment. Persistent delirium is also a risk factor for cognitive impairment, emergency visits, hospitalization, or death (Cole et al. 2017; Pereira et al. 2021). As described in Statement 1, several structured assessments can be used to identify delirium and its persistence after discharge.

Even when delirium has resolved, discharge from the hospital is associated with significant risk of readmission, nursing facility placement, and mortality (Rahman and Byatt 2021). Ongoing assessments of cognitive and physical functioning are recommended after hospital discharge

(Guthrie et al. 2018; Mikkelsen et al. 2020). Risks of persistent cognitive impairment are increased in patients who have had delirium (Cole and McCusker 2016; Goldberg et al. 2020; Pandharipande et al. 2013; Pereira et al. 2021; van den Boogaard et al. 2012), and cognitive (Kunicki et al. 2023) and functional decline and disability (Wilson et al. 2020) are also increased compared with hospitalized patients without delirium. Bedside assessments of cognitive function such as the MoCA (Nasreddine et al. 2005), the MMSE (Folstein et al. 1975, 2010), and the Saint Louis University Mental Status (SLUMS; Cummings-Vaughn et al. 2014; Tariq et al. 2006) are often used for assessing cognitive domains. For rating of functioning, the World Health Organization Disability Assessment Schedule 2.0 (WHODAS 2.0) is available in a 36-item version that requires about 20 minutes to complete, as well as a 12-item version, which requires about 5 minutes to complete (American Psychiatric Association 2022; World Health Organization 2010). In addition to providing scores for cognition, mobility, self-care, getting along with people, and life activities (household and work), the WHODAS 2.0 is available in multiple languages and can be completed by the patient, a proxy, or an interviewer either in person or by phone (World Health Organization 2010).

In addition to a need for postdischarge assessment of cognition, other long-term consequences of delirium that warrant assessment during follow-up may include anxiety, depression, PTSD, and impairments in quality of life (Bolton et al. 2021; Guthrie et al. 2018; Mikkelsen et al. 2020; Ramnarain et al. 2023; Weidman et al. 2022; Wilson et al. 2020; Wolters et al. 2016). Rates of PTSD have been best studied in ICU patients but appear to be increased in patients with delirium (Battle et al. 2017; Bolton et al. 2021; Bulic et al. 2020; Friberg et al. 2024; Griffin et al. 2023; Rengel et al. 2021). Examples of scales that can be used to assess for posttraumatic stress symptoms and PTSD include the Impact of Event Scale—Revised (Creamer et al. 2003) and the PTSD Checklist for DSM-5 (PCL-5; Blevins et al. 2015), respectively. Rates of anxiety and depression also appear to be increased after critical care hospitalization but have been less well studied in patients with delirium (Bolton et al. 2021; Ramnarain et al. 2023; Rengel et al. 2021; Wilson et al. 2020). Screening for depression and anxiety can be done with scales such as the Patient Health Questionnaire-9 (PHQ-9; Kroenke et al. 2001), the Geriatric Depression Scale (GDS; Mitchell et al. 2010; Sheikh and Yesavage 1986; Yesavage et al. 1982–1983), the Generalized Anxiety Disorder Scale (GAD-7; Spitzer et al. 2006), or the Hospital Anxiety and Depression Scale (Zigmond and Snaith 1983). For individuals who are able to complete a self-report measure, quality of life can be assessed with the World Health Organization Quality of Life BREF (WHOQOL-BREF; The WHOQOL Group 1998a), which has strong psychometric properties (Grassi et al. 2020; The WHOQOL Group 1998a, 1998b). Other measures are also available for assessing cognition, functioning, and quality of life (Giedzinska and Wilson 2023; Rush et al. 2008), although interventions during follow-up to improve outcomes have been limited (Schofield-Robinson et al. 2018).

It is imperative that patients, caregivers, and family members receive education about delirium following discharge to home; however, such information is often not provided (Chuen et al. 2021; Meyer et al. 2023). Patients often report feeling distressed while delirious, and some have delusional ideas about their experiences and persistent fears after hospital discharge (Breitbart et al. 2002; Gaete Ortega et al. 2020). Family members and other caregivers are also interested in receiving information about delirium, including symptoms and causes of delirium, as well as ways to help in managing it (Meyer et al. 2023; Shrestha and Fick 2020). The fluctuating presentation of delirium, as well as symptoms such as hallucinations, delusions, and agitation, may be concerning to observe. Family members and caregivers can benefit from transparent discussions of these experiences and associated anxiety or emotional distress (Assa et al. 2021; Breitbart et al. 2002; Meyer et al. 2023).

After discharge, formal or informal caregivers may be needed to help patients adhere to postdischarge medical plans (e.g., assist with remembering to take medication), including physical rehabilitation, and in some instances to assist with activities of daily living (O'Rourke et al. 2021; Rengel et al. 2021). Consequently, these caregivers will be in a good position to recognize changes in symptoms and functioning and ensure that patients receive quick access to health care if they experience physical symptoms or reductions in functioning (Carbone and Gugliucci 2015). Studies suggest that, when properly educated, family members and other caregivers can be reliable informants and can accurately identify and describe in detail the patient's delirium symptoms (Shrestha and Fick 2020), which can be useful in identifying persistence or recurrence of delirium. For these reasons, providing patients, families, and other caregivers with information about delirium may help diminish residual emotional effects of the delirium experience and can enhance their ability to partner in care after discharge (J. Lee et al. 2023; Meyer et al. 2023).

Areas for Further Research

As with any psychiatric disorder, multiple issues related to delirium would benefit from further research. These include research topics such as the following:

Screening and Assessment

- Determine whether patient characteristics and factors that confer risk for delirium can be used to identify patients at a high likelihood of developing delirium who could benefit from early intervention.
- Determine whether patterns of subsyndromal symptoms or motor symptoms, either alone or in combination with patient characteristics and delirium risk factors, can be used to identify patients at a high likelihood of developing delirium who could benefit from early intervention.
- Determine whether additional rating scales need to be developed for delirium identification, diagnosis, or rating of severity that are brief to administer, require limited training, and are valid and reliable among a broad range of settings (e.g., critical care, other hospital units, ambulatory practice, skilled nursing facilities), ages, genders, cultures, languages, social determinants of health, symptom patterns (e.g., hyperactive vs. hypoactive), and underlying pathophysiologies.
- Identify methods that will allow refinement of clinical assessment and delirium "phenotyping" by using physiological monitoring (e.g., electroencephalogram, electrocardiogram), wearable technology, predictive modeling, and large-scale data analytics.

Treatment

- Identify subtypes of delirium that would require distinct treatment approaches to achieve optimal patient outcomes.
- Identify significant symptoms (e.g., agitation, hallucinations), co-occurring conditions (e.g., coronavirus SARS-CoV-2 disease 2019, substance-related disorders, other psychiatric disorders), biomarkers, and other factors that can help in individualizing treatment selection, frequency, and duration to achieve optimal patient outcomes.
- Identify approaches to individualizing treatment selection and delivery to optimize outcomes among a broad range of settings (e.g., critical care, other hospital units, ambulatory practice, skilled nursing facilities), ages, genders, cultures, languages, social determinants of health, symptom patterns (e.g., hyperactive vs. hypoactive), co-occurring disorders (e.g., dementia, intellectual disabilities), and underlying pathophysiologies.
- Obtain additional evidence on novel or existing pharmacotherapies (e.g., cholinesterase inhibitors; α-adrenergic agents) in the treatment of delirium.
- Obtain additional evidence on novel or existing pharmacotherapies (e.g., dexmedetomidine, antipsychotic agents) in the treatment of specific symptoms of delirium (e.g., agitation, aggression, psychosis).

- Identify the specific elements of multicomponent interventions that have the greatest effect on specific delirium outcomes, as well as the intervention "dose" (e.g., time spent, frequency, consistency of use) and implementation features (e.g., workflows, staffing) that are needed for benefits to occur.
- Obtain additional evidence on novel or existing nonpharmacological interventions (e.g., rehabilitative therapies) in the treatment of delirium or specific symptoms of delirium (e.g., agitation, aggression, psychosis).
- Identify the treatment elements and approaches to care and communication that are viewed as most and least helpful by individuals who have recovered from delirium and by their family members or other caregivers.
- Identify optimal approaches to providing patient, family, and other caregivers education and support when delirium is present and after it has resolved.
- Identify optimal approaches to engaging family and other caregivers in caring for individuals with delirium or at risk for delirium.

Systems of Care

- Identify approaches to adapting workflows and models of care delivery to improve the use of best practices and reduce inequities in the care of individuals with delirium among a broad range of settings (e.g., independent living, ambulatory practice, critical care, other hospital units, skilled nursing facilities).
- Identify approaches to adapting workflows and models of care delivery to reduce biases (including race/ethnicity and preferred language) in delirium identification (e.g., hypoactive vs. hyperactive subtype, preexisting cognitive impairment or frailty) and use of interventions (e.g., physical restraints, psychotropic medication).
- Identify optimal approaches to longitudinal monitoring and follow-up care of patients with delirium after transitioning from an acute care setting.

Study Design Considerations

In addition to these specific topics that would benefit from additional research, the ability to draw clinically meaningful conclusions from research would be augmented by improvements in the design of studies. Current evidence on delirium has been limited by several factors:

- Studies are not always registered (e.g., in https://ClinicalTrials.gov) with the prespecification of outcomes of interest.
- Study designs do not typically fulfill all elements to achieve a low risk of study bias or do not provide sufficient information to determine the degree of study bias with accuracy (e.g., randomization and blinding procedures, statistical approaches for missing data).
- Procedures for the screening and assessment of delirium have not always been well described in terms of scale administration, training of raters, and inter- and intrarater reliability.
- Sample sizes are often small, limiting the ability to stratify analyses or achieve the statistical power to detect differences due to intervention effects.
- Sample characteristics have been limited in their breadth (e.g., older individuals, critical care or medical inpatients) and ascertainment approaches (e.g., particular units, postoperative patients with cardiac or orthopedic procedures).
- Sample characteristics are not well described (e.g., age; gender; race/ethnicity; preferred language; hypoactive vs. hyperactive delirium; levels of consciousness and arousal; underlying

pathophysiology; delirium severity; presence or absence of specific risk factors, diagnostic criteria exclusions, or preexisting cognitive impairment).

- Samples have not always excluded comatose patients or patients with preexisting delirium.
- Interventions for prevention and treatment of delirium have varied in study design and treatment implementation (e.g., variable use of nonpharmacological approaches; differences in dose, timing, frequency, and route of medication administration).
- Outcomes of medication studies have not distinguished between effects on delirium, per se, and reductions in hyperactivity due to sedation.
- Information on harms, including in nonpharmacological studies, typically has not been collected in a systematic fashion.
- Follow-up duration is often brief, and outcomes have focused on delirium incidence, delirium duration, length of stay (ICU or hospital), or readmission rates, with minimal attention to specific symptoms (e.g., agitation, aggression, hallucinations) or short- and long-term functional outcomes.

Guideline Development Process

This guideline was developed using a process intended to meet the standards of the Institute of Medicine (2011; now known as the National Academy of Medicine). The process is fully described in a document available on the APA website at: www.psychiatry.org/psychiatrists/practice/clinical-practice-guidelines/guideline-development-process. Key aspects of the process for developing the guideline statements are also described in the "Introduction" (see section "Rating the Strengths of Guideline Statements and Supporting Research Evidence").

Management of Potential Conflicts of Interest

Members of the Guideline Writing Group (GWG) are required to disclose all potential conflicts of interest before appointment, before and during guideline development, and on publication. If any potential conflicts are found or disclosed during the guideline development process, the member must recuse themself from any related discussion and voting on a related recommendation. The members of both the GWG and the Systematic Review Group (SRG) reported no conflicts of interest. The "Disclosures" section includes more detailed disclosure information for each GWG and SRG member involved in the guideline's development.

Guideline Writing Group Composition

In addition to the chair of the GWG (C.C.), the GWG was initially composed of five psychiatrists with general research and clinical expertise (I.A., R.B., J.I.E., M.J.-T., A.S.) and one psychiatrist with general research and clinical expertise who is also board certified in family medicine (T.H.). This non-topic-specific group was intended to provide diverse and balanced views on the guideline topic to minimize potential bias. Two psychiatrists (J.L.L., M.A.O.), one internist (M.M.), and one critical care nursing researcher (M.C.B.) were added to provide subject matter expertise in delirium. One fellow (J.M.T.) was involved in the guideline development process. The vice-chair of the GWG (L.J.F.) provided methodological expertise on topics such as appraising the strength of research evidence. The GWG was also diverse and balanced with respect to other characteristics, such as geographic location and demographic background. The draft was distributed to a wide range of professional organizations and patient and family advocacy groups to solicit comments.

Systematic Review Methodology

This guideline is based on a systematic search of available research evidence conducted by the Pacific Northwest Evidence-Based Practice Center. The methods for this systematic review followed the Agency for Healthcare Research and Quality (AHRQ) *Methods Guide for Effectiveness and Comparative Effectiveness Reviews* (available at: https://effectivehealthcare.ahrq.gov/products/collections/cer-methods-guide).

Searches were conducted in Ovid, MEDLINE, PsycINFO, EMBASE, Cochrane Central Register of Controlled Trials, and Cochrane Database of Systematic Reviews from database inception through October 2020 (as described in Appendix B, Tables B-1 through B-6) to identify studies eligible for this review, according to preestablished criteria listed in Appendix B, Table B-7, and summarized in Table 10. An updated search using the same criteria spanned the period from October 2020 through July 9, 2021. Studies were restricted to adults (age 18 years and older) who were at risk for delirium, had a clinical diagnosis of delirium, or met DSM criteria for delirium. Included studies were restricted to English-language articles and interventions that were available in the United States. Observational studies with at least 50 participants were included only if inadequate evidence was found in RCTs for primary outcomes on any Key Questions (see Appendix A).

As shown in Appendix B, Figure B-1, the systematic review retrieved 12,102 articles, of which 10,903 were excluded based on the screening of titles and abstracts. The full text of the remaining 1,199 articles was reviewed, and 277 articles met the inclusion criteria, with 204 articles related to prevention of delirium, 51 articles related to treatment, and 12 articles related to both prevention and treatment. The updated search yielded an additional 912 articles, of which 805 were excluded based on title and abstract screening. Of the remaining 107 full-text articles that were reviewed, 37 articles met the inclusion criteria, with 31 articles related to prevention of delirium, 4 articles related to treatment, and 2 articles related to both prevention and treatment. For both the initial and the updated searches, titles and abstracts were screened by an initial reviewer, and excluded articles were screened by a second reviewer. Full-text review was conducted in duplicate. Any discrepant determinations in title/abstract or full-text review were resolved by consensus with input included from a third individual if consensus could not be reached. Available guidelines from other organizations also were reviewed (Aldecoa et al. 2017; American College of Emergency

TABLE 10 Criteria for populations, interventions, comparisons, and outcomes of eligible studies of delirium

	Include	Exclude
Populations	Adults (age 18 years and older) at risk for delirium or with delirium, including those on palliative care and at end of life	Children and adolescents (younger than 18 years)
Interventions	Medication interventions (e.g., antipsychotics, cholinesterase inhibitors, sedatives, hypnotics, analgesics, melatonin, over-the-counter medications, complementary and alternative medicine) and nonmedication interventions (e.g., environmental, light therapy, pain management, psychosocial interventions, reduction of unnecessary medications)	No intervention
Comparisons	Placebo, no intervention (usual care), other medication interventions, other nonmedication interventions, and different doses, frequencies, or intensities of interventions	No comparison
Outcomes	Incidence and severity of delirium, frequency of delirium episodes, duration of delirium, agitation, readmission or admission to hospital, quality of life, caregiver burden, rescue medication use, length of stay in hospital or ICU, mortality, adverse events	None
Duration	Any duration	None
Settings	Any setting, including inpatient, hospice, and nursing homes	None
Study designs	RCTs, observational studies with 50 or more participants, nonrandomized clinical studies with a comparator; best evidence approach	Uncontrolled, observational study with no comparator

Note. ICU=intensive care unit; RCT=randomized controlled trial.

Physicians 2014; American Geriatrics Society Expert Panel on Postoperative Delirium in Older Adults 2015; American Psychiatric Association 1999; BC Centre for Palliative Care 2017a, 2017b; Bush et al. 2018; Cancer Care Ontario 2010; Chow et al. 2012; Danish Health Authority 2021; Devlin et al. 2018; Gage and Hogan 2014; Martin et al. 2010; Mohanty et al. 2016; National Institute for Health and Care Excellence 2023; Potter et al. 2006; Registered Nurses' Association of Ontario 2016; Scottish Intercollegiate Guidelines Network 2019; Tropea et al. 2008; see Appendix F).

Data were abstracted from included studies into evidence tables (see Appendix D), including study and patient characteristics and study results, with data verified for accuracy and completeness by a second team member. Predefined criteria were used to assess the risk of bias of included trials. RCTs were assessed based on criteria established in the *Cochrane Handbook for Systematic Reviews of Interventions* (Furlan et al. 2015; Higgins et al. 2023), with observational studies assessed using criteria developed by the U.S. Preventive Services Task Force (Harris et al. 2001). Two team members independently assessed the risk of bias and assigned an overall rating of low, moderate, or high risk of bias, with disagreements resolved by consensus. Risk of bias ratings are included in evidence tables (see Appendix D), with specific factors contributing to the risk of bias for each study shown in Appendix E.

Evidence was analyzed according to Key Questions, using both qualitative (narrative) and, when possible, quantitative (meta-analysis) methods. In both approaches, medication studies were grouped by setting (e.g., surgical, ICU, general inpatient), and nonmedication studies were grouped by intervention type (single component vs. multicomponent). For medication studies, within each setting, medications of the same general class were assessed together. For outcomes of delirium incidence, severity, and duration; ICU and hospital length of stay; and mortality, meta-analyses were conducted when at least two studies reported the same outcome. Study quality and heterogeneity among studies (in design, patient population, interventions, and outcomes) were also considered in determining whether to conduct meta-analyses. A detailed description of meta-analytic methods is provided in Appendix B. In addition, the Pacific Northwest Evidence-Based Practice Center graded primary outcome-intervention pairs for delirium incidence, severity, and duration and adverse events. Using AHRQ methods (Berkman et al. 2015), the body of research evidence was categorized as having high, moderate, or low strength, reflecting the confidence or certainty in the findings (see Appendix B, Table B-8). Bodies of research evidence with inadequate evidence were judged to be insufficient to draw conclusions. In addition, the magnitudes of effects were summarized according to thresholds of little to no difference and small, moderate, or large effects, regardless of the statistical significance of the differences (see Appendix B, Table B-9).

External Review

This guideline was made available for review in January–March 2024 by the APA membership, scientific and clinical experts, allied organizations, and the public. In addition, some patient advocacy organizations were invited for input. Twenty-one individuals, two councils of the APA, and nine other organizations submitted comments on this guideline (see the section "Individuals and Organizations That Submitted Comments" for a list of the names). The chair and vice-chair of the GWG reviewed and addressed all comments received; the GWG reviewed substantive issues.

Funding and Approval

This guideline development project was funded and supported by the APA without any involvement of industry or external funding. The guideline was submitted to the APA Assembly and APA Board of Trustees and approved on October 11, 2024, and November 20, 2024, respectively.

References

Abilify (aripiprazole) [prescribing information]. Rockville, MD, Otsuka America Pharmaceutical Inc, November 2022

Adeola M, Azad R, Kassie GM, et al: Multicomponent interventions reduce high-risk medications for delirium in hospitalized older adults. J Am Geriatr Soc 66(8):1638–1645, 2018 30035315

Agboola IK, Coupet E Jr, Wong AH: "The coats that we can take off and the ones we can't": the role of trauma-informed care on race and bias during agitation in the emergency department. Ann Emerg Med 77(5):493–498, 2021 33579587

Agency for Healthcare Research and Quality: Methods Guide for Effectiveness and Comparative Effectiveness Reviews (AHRQ Publ No 10(14)-EHC063-EF). Rockville, MD, Agency for Healthcare Research and Quality, January 2014. Available at: https://effectivehealthcare.ahrq.gov/sites/default/files/pdf/cer-methods-guide_overview.pdf. Accessed February 15, 2017.

Akamine Y, Yasui-Furukori N, Ieiri I, et al: Psychotropic drug-drug interactions involving P-glycoprotein. CNS Drugs 26(11):959–973, 2012 23023659

Aldecoa C, Bettelli G, Bilotta F, et al: European Society of Anaesthesiology evidence-based and consensus-based guideline on postoperative delirium. Eur J Anaesthesiol 34(4):192–214, 2017 28187050

Aldwikat RK, Manias E, Tomlinson E, et al: Delirium screening tools in the post-anaesthetic care unit: a systematic review and meta-analysis. Aging Clin Exp Res 34(6):1225–1235, 2022 34981431

Ali MA, Hashmi M, Ahmed W, et al: Incidence and risk factors of delirium in surgical intensive care unit. Trauma Surg Acute Care Open 6(1):e000564, 2021 33748426

Alper K, Schwartz KA, Kolts RL, et al: Seizure incidence in psychopharmacological clinical trials: an analysis of Food and Drug Administration (FDA) summary basis of approval reports. Biol Psychiatry 62(4):345–354, 2007 17223086

American College of Emergency Physicians; American Geriatrics Society; Emergency Nurses Association; Society for Academic Emergency Medicine; Geriatric Emergency Department Guidelines Task Force: Geriatric emergency department guidelines. Ann Emerg Med 63(5):e7–e25, 2014 24746437

American College of Surgeons: Optimal Resources for Geriatric Surgery: 2019 Standards. Chicago, IL, American College of Surgeons, 2019. Available at: https://www.facs.org/media/yldfbgwz/optimal-resources-for-geriatric-surgery-2019-standards.pdf. Accessed July 20, 2024.

American Geriatrics Society Beers Criteria® Update Expert Panel: American Geriatrics Society 2023 updated AGS Beers Criteria® for potentially inappropriate medication use in older adults. J Am Geriatr Soc 71(7):2052–2081, 2023 37139824

American Geriatrics Society Expert Panel on Postoperative Delirium in Older Adults: American Geriatrics Society abstracted clinical practice guideline for postoperative delirium in older adults. J Am Geriatr Soc 63(1):142–150, 2015 25495432

American Psychiatric Association: Diagnostic and Statistical Manual of Mental Disorders, 3rd Edition, Revised. Washington, DC, American Psychiatric Association, 1987

American Psychiatric Association: Diagnostic and Statistical Manual of Mental Disorders, 4th Edition. Washington, DC, American Psychiatric Association, 1994

American Psychiatric Association: Practice guideline for the treatment of patients with delirium. Am J Psychiatry 156(5 Suppl):1–20, 1999 10327941

American Psychiatric Association: Diagnostic and Statistical Manual of Mental Disorders, 5th Edition. Arlington, VA, American Psychiatric Association, 2013

American Psychiatric Association: The American Psychiatric Association Practice Guideline on the Use of Antipsychotics to Treat Agitation or Psychosis in Patients With Dementia. Arlington, VA, American Psychiatric Association, 2016

American Psychiatric Association: The American Psychiatric Association Practice Guideline for the Treatment of Patients With Schizophrenia, 3rd Edition. Washington, DC, American Psychiatric Association, 2021

American Psychiatric Association: Diagnostic and Statistical Manual of Mental Disorders, 5th Edition, Text Revision. Washington, DC, American Psychiatric Association, 2022

American Society of Addiction Medicine: The Joint Clinical Practice Guideline on Benzodiazepine Tapering: Considerations When Benzodiazepine Risks Outweigh Benefits. 2025. Available at: https://www.asam.org/quality-care/clinical-guidelines/benzodiazepine-tapering. Accessed April 7, 2025.

Anand A, Cheng M, Ibitoye T, et al: Positive scores on the 4AT delirium assessment tool at hospital admission are linked to mortality, length of stay and home time: two-centre study of 82,770 emergency admissions. Age Ageing 51(3):afac051, 2022 35292792

Andersen-Ranberg NC, Poulsen LM, Perner A, et al; AID-ICU Trial Group: Haloperidol for the treatment of delirium in ICU patients. N Engl J Med 387(26):2425–2435, 2022 36286254

Andersen-Ranberg NC, Barbateskovic M, Perner A, et al: Haloperidol for the treatment of delirium in critically ill patients: an updated systematic review with meta-analysis and trial sequential analysis. Crit Care 27(1):329, 2023a 37633991

Andersen-Ranberg NC, Poulsen LM, Perner A, et al: Haloperidol vs. placebo for the treatment of delirium in ICU patients: a pre-planned, secondary Bayesian analysis of the AID-ICU trial. Intensive Care Med 49(4):411–420, 2023b 36971791

Andrews JC, Schünemann HJ, Oxman AD, et al: GRADE guidelines: 15. Going from evidence to recommendation-determinants of a recommendation's direction and strength. J Clin Epidemiol 66(7):726–735, 2013 23570745

Andrews PS, Wang S, Perkins AJ, et al: Relationship between intensive care unit delirium severity and 2-year mortality and health care utilization. Am J Crit Care 29(4):311–317, 2020 32607574

Appiani FJ, Duarte JM, Sauré M, et al: Catatonia and delirium: assessment of comorbidity, prevalence, and therapeutic response in medically ill inpatients from a university hospital. J Clin Psychopharmacol 43(1):55–59, 2023 36584250

Arias F, Alegria M, Kind AJ, et al: A framework of social determinants of health for delirium tailored to older adults. J Am Geriatr Soc 70(1):235–242, 2022 34693992

Aripiprazole orally disintegrating tablets [prescribing information]. Bridgewater, NJ, Alembic Pharmaceuticals, November 2018

Aripiprazole solution [prescribing information]. Weston, FL, Apotex, November 2016

Armstrong SC, Cozza KL, Sandson NB: Six patterns of drug-drug interactions. Psychosomatics 44(3):255–258, 2003 12724509

Assa AH, Wicks MN, Umberger RA: Family caregivers' experience of patients with delirium in critical care units: a state-of-the-science integrative review. Am J Crit Care 30(6):471–478, 2021 34719705

Awan OM, Buhr RG, Kamdar BB: Factors influencing CAM-ICU documentation and inappropriate "Unable to Assess" responses. Am J Crit Care 30(6):e99–e107, 2021 34719712

Bahji A, Bach P, Danilewitz M, et al: Comparative efficacy and safety of pharmacotherapies for alcohol withdrawal: a systematic review and network meta-analysis. Addiction 117(10):2591–2601, 2022 35194860

Balas MC, Tan A, Pun BT, et al: Effects of a national quality improvement collaborative on ABCDEF bundle implementation. Am J Crit Care 31(1):54–64, 2022 34972842

Balshem H, Helfand M, Schünemann HJ, et al: GRADE guidelines: 3. Rating the quality of evidence. J Clin Epidemiol 64(4):401–406, 2011 21208779

Barnes-Daly MA, Phillips G, Ely EW: Improving hospital survival and reducing brain dysfunction at seven California community hospitals: implementing PAD guidelines via the ABCDEF bundle in 6,064 patients. Crit Care Med 45(2):171–178, 2017 27861180

Basciotta M, Zhou W, Ngo L, et al: Antipsychotics and the risk of mortality or cardiopulmonary arrest in hospitalized adults. J Am Geriatr Soc 68(3):544–550, 2020 31743435

Battle CE, James K, Bromfield T, et al: Predictors of post-traumatic stress disorder following critical illness: a mixed methods study. J Intensive Care Soc 18(4):289–293, 2017 29123558

BC Centre for Palliative Care: B.C. Inter-professional Palliative Symptom Management Guidelines. New Westminster, BC, Canada, BC Centre for Palliative Care, 2017a. Available at: https://bc-cpc.ca/wp-content/uploads/2018/09/SMGs-interactive-final-Nov-30-compressed.pdf. Accessed December 5, 2023.

BC Centre for Palliative Care: Palliative Care for the Patient With Incurable Cancer or Advanced Disease, Part 2: Pain and Symptom Management. New Westminster, BC, Canada, BC Centre for Palliative Care, 2017b. Available at: https://www2.gov.bc.ca/assets/gov/health/practitioner-pro/bc-guidelines/palliative2.pdf. Accessed December 5, 2023.

Beach SR, Gross AF, Hartney KE, et al: Intravenous haloperidol: a systematic review of side effects and recommendations for clinical use. Gen Hosp Psychiatry 67:42–50, 2020 32979582

Béland E, Nadeau A, Carmichael PH, et al: Predictors of delirium in older patients at the emergency department: a prospective multicentre derivation study. CJEM 23(3):330–336, 2021 33959922

Bellelli G, Morandi A, Davis DH, et al: Validation of the 4AT, a new instrument for rapid delirium screening: a study in 234 hospitalised older people. Age Ageing 43(4):496–502, 2014 24590568

Ber J, Wiczling P, Hołysz M, et al: Population pharmacokinetic model of dexmedetomidine in a heterogeneous group of patients. J Clin Pharmacol 60(11):1461–1473, 2020 32500578

Bergeron N, Dubois MJ, Dumont M, et al: Intensive Care Delirium Screening Checklist: evaluation of a new screening tool. Intensive Care Med 27(5):859–864, 2001 11430542

Bergl PA: At baseline. N Engl J Med 380(19):1792–1793, 2019 31067368

Berkman ND, Lohr KN, Ansari MT, et al: Grading the strength of a body of evidence when assessing health care interventions: an EPC update. J Clin Epidemiol 68(11):1312–1324, 2015 25721570

Berzlanovich AM, Schöpfer J, Keil W: Deaths due to physical restraint. Dtsch Arztebl Int 109(3):27–32, 2012 22334818

Bhattacharyya S, Darby RR, Raibagkar P, et al: Antibiotic-associated encephalopathy. Neurology 86(10):963–971, 2016 26888997

Bjerre Real C, Dhawan V, Sharma M, et al: Delirium in critically ill cancer patients with COVID-19. J Acad Consult Liaison Psychiatry 63(6):539–547, 2022 35660676

Blevins CA, Weathers FW, Davis MT, et al: The Posttraumatic Stress Disorder Checklist for DSM-5 (PCL-5): development and initial psychometric evaluation. J Trauma Stress 28(6):489–498, 2015 26606250

Bloomfield HE, Greer N, Linsky AM, et al: Deprescribing for community-dwelling older adults: a systematic review and meta-analysis. J Gen Intern Med 35(11):3323–3332, 2020 32820421

Boehm LM, Jones AC, Selim AA, et al: Delirium-related distress in the ICU: a qualitative meta-synthesis of patient and family perspectives and experiences. Int J Nurs Stud 122:104030, 2021 34343884

Bolton C, Thilges S, Lane C, et al: Post-traumatic stress disorder following acute delirium. J Clin Psychol Med Settings 28(1):31–39, 2021 31823162

Boltz M, BeLue R, Resnick B, et al: Disparities in physical and psychological symptoms in hospitalized African American and White persons with dementia. J Aging Health 33(5-6):340–349, 2021 33371763

Boncyk CS, Farrin E, Stollings JL, et al: Pharmacologic management of intensive care unit delirium: clinical prescribing practices and outcomes in more than 8500 patient encounters. Anesth Analg 133(3):713–722, 2021 33433117

Bowman EML, Brummel NE, Caplan GA, et al: Advancing specificity in delirium: the delirium subtyping initiative. Alzheimers Dement 20(1):183–194, 2024 37522255
Bradley EH, Schlesinger M, Webster TR, et al: Translating research into clinical practice: making change happen. J Am Geriatr Soc 52(11):1875–1882, 2004 15507065
Bradley EH, Webster TR, Schlesinger M, et al: Patterns of diffusion of evidence-based clinical programmes: a case study of the Hospital Elder Life Program. Qual Saf Health Care 15(5):334–338, 2006 17074869
Bramley P, McArthur K, Blayney A, et al: Risk factors for postoperative delirium: an umbrella review of systematic reviews. Int J Surg 93:106063, 2021 34411752
Breitbart W, Rosenfeld B, Roth A, et al: The Memorial Delirium Assessment Scale. J Pain Symptom Manage 13(3):128–137, 1997 9114631
Breitbart W, Gibson C, Tremblay A: The delirium experience: delirium recall and delirium-related distress in hospitalized patients with cancer, their spouses/caregivers, and their nurses. Psychosomatics 43(3):183–194, 2002 12075033
Brill MJ, van Rongen A, van Dongen EP, et al: The pharmacokinetics of the CYP3A substrate midazolam in morbidly obese patients before and one year after bariatric surgery. Pharm Res 32(12):3927–3936, 2015 26202517
Brito JP, Domecq JP, Murad MH, et al: The Endocrine Society guidelines: when the confidence cart goes before the evidence horse. J Clin Endocrinol Metab 98(8):3246–3252, 2013 23783104
Brockman A, Krupp A, Bach C, et al: Clinicians' perceptions on implementation strategies used to facilitate ABCDEF bundle adoption: a multicenter survey. Heart Lung 62:108–115, 2023 37399777
Brown JC, Querubin JA, Ding L, et al: Improving ABCDEF bundle compliance and clinical outcomes in the ICU: randomized control trial to assess the impact of performance measurement, feedback, and data literacy training. Crit Care Explor 4(4):e0679, 2022 35474653
Bulic D, Bennett M, Georgousopoulou EN, et al: Cognitive and psychosocial outcomes of mechanically ventilated intensive care patients with and without delirium. Ann Intensive Care 10(1):104, 2020 32748298
Buljac-Samardzic M, Doekhie KD, van Wijngaarden JDH: Interventions to improve team effectiveness within health care: a systematic review of the past decade. Hum Resour Health 18(1):2, 2020 31915007
Burry LD, Bell CM, Hill A, et al: New and persistent sedative prescriptions among older adults following a critical illness: a population-based cohort study. Chest 163(6):1425–1436, 2023 36610663
Burton JK, Craig L, Yong SQ, et al: Non-pharmacological interventions for preventing delirium in hospitalised non-ICU patients. Cochrane Database Syst Rev 11:Cd013307, 2021a 34826144
Burton JK, Fearon P, Noel-Storr AH, et al: Informant Questionnaire on Cognitive Decline in the Elderly (IQCODE) for the detection of dementia within a secondary care setting. Cochrane Database Syst Rev 7(7):CD010772, 2021b 34278561
Burton JK, Stott DJ, McShane R, et al: Informant Questionnaire on Cognitive Decline in the Elderly (IQCODE) for the early detection of dementia across a variety of healthcare settings. Cochrane Database Syst Rev 7(7):CD011333, 2021c 34275145
Bush SH, Bruera E: The assessment and management of delirium in cancer patients. Oncologist 14(10):1039–1049, 2009 19808772
Bush SH, Tierney S, Lawlor PG: Clinical assessment and management of delirium in the palliative care setting. Drugs 77(15):1623–1643, 2017 28864877
Bush SH, Lawlor PG, Ryan K, et al; ESMO Guidelines Committee: Delirium in adult cancer patients: ESMO Clinical Practice Guidelines. Ann Oncol 29(Suppl 4):iv143–iv165, 2018 29992308
Butcher JD, Smith MC, Roberts L, et al: Utility of head computed tomography for older adults with suspected delirium in the emergency department: a retrospective observational study. Acad Emerg Med 30(1):16–22, 2023 36478487
Cai S, Li J, Gao J, et al: Prediction models for postoperative delirium after cardiac surgery: systematic review and critical appraisal. Int J Nurs Stud 136:104340, 2022 36208541
California Senate Bill No 1254: SB-1254 Hospital Pharmacies: Medication Profiles or Lists for High-Risk Patients. California Legislative Information, Approved September 22, 2018. Available at: https://leginfo.legislature.ca.gov/faces/billNavClient.xhtml?bill_id=201720180SB1254. Accessed August 8, 2023.
Campbell NL, Cantor BB, Hui SL, et al: Race and documentation of cognitive impairment in hospitalized older adults. J Am Geriatr Soc 62(3):506–511, 2014 24576177
Cancer Care Ontario: Cancer Care Ontario's Symptom Management Guide-to-Practice: Delirium. Toronto, ON, Canada, Cancer Care Ontario, August 2010. Available at: https://www.cancercareontario.ca/en/symptom-management/3136. Accessed December 5, 2023.
Caplan GA, Teodorczuk A, Streatfeild J, et al: The financial and social costs of delirium. Eur Geriatr Med 11(1):105–112, 2020 32297239
Caravella RA, Ying P, Siegel C, et al: Quality improvement framework to examine health care disparities in behavioral emergency management in the inpatient medical setting: a consultation-liaison psychiatry health equity project. J Acad Consult Liaison Psychiatry 64(4):322–331, 2023 37060945
Carbone MK, Gugliucci MR: Delirium and the family caregiver: the need for evidence-based education interventions. Gerontologist 55(3):345–352, 2015 24847844
Caroff SN, Watson CB, Rosenberg H: Drug-induced hyperthermic syndromes in psychiatry. Clin Psychopharmacol Neurosci 19(1):1–11, 2021 33508784
Carpenter CR, Hammouda N, Linton EA, et al; GEAR Network: Delirium prevention, detection, and treatment in emergency medicine settings: a geriatric emergency care applied research (GEAR) network scoping review and consensus statement. Acad Emerg Med 28(1):19–35, 2021 33135274
Carreras Tartak JA, Brisbon N, Wilkie S, et al: Racial and ethnic disparities in emergency department restraint use: a multicenter retrospective analysis. Acad Emerg Med 28(9):957–965, 2021 34533261

Centers for Disease Control and Prevention: Prescription Drug Monitoring Programs (PDMPs). Atlanta, GA, Centers for Disease Control and Prevention, 2021. Available at: https://www.cdc.gov/drugoverdose/pdmp/index.html. Accessed July 12, 2023.
Centers for Medicare & Medicaid Services: A Practical Guide to Implementing the National CLAS Standards: For Racial, Ethnic and Linguistic Minorities, People With Disabilities and Sexual and Gender Minorities. Baltimore, MD, Centers for Medicare & Medicaid Services, December 2016. Available at: https://lgbtagingcenter.org/wp-content/uploads/2024/06/CLAS-Toolkit-12-7-16.pdf. Accessed July 21, 2024.
Ceschi A, Noseda R, Pironi M, et al: Effect of medication reconciliation at hospital admission on 30-day returns to hospital: a randomized clinical trial. JAMA Netw Open 4(9):e2124672, 2021 34529065
Chaiwat O, Chanidnuan M, Pancharoen W, et al: Postoperative delirium in critically ill surgical patients: incidence, risk factors, and predictive scores. BMC Anesthesiol 19(1):39, 2019 30894129
Champion C, Novais T, Dorey JM, et al: Paradoxical reactions to benzodiazepines in the elderly [in French]. Geriatr Psychol Neuropsychiatr Vieil 19(3):305–312, 2021 34526288
Chen F, Liu L, Wang Y, et al: Delirium prevalence in geriatric emergency department patients: a systematic review and meta-analysis. Am J Emerg Med 59:121–128, 2022 35841845
Chen H, Mo L, Hu H, et al: Risk factors of postoperative delirium after cardiac surgery: a meta-analysis. J Cardiothorac Surg 16(1):113, 2021 33902644
Chen TJ, Traynor V, Wang AY, et al: Comparative effectiveness of non-pharmacological interventions for preventing delirium in critically ill adults: a systematic review and network meta-analysis. Int J Nurs Stud 131:104239, 2022 35468538
Chlorpromazine hydrochloride concentrate [prescribing information]. Princeton, NJ, Sandoz, Inc, January 2023
Chlorpromazine hydrochloride injection [prescribing information]. East Windsor, NJ, Eugia US, LLC, June 2023
Chlorpromazine hydrochloride tablets [prescribing information]. Bedminster, NJ, Alembic Pharmaceuticals, Inc, April 2024
Chow WB, Rosenthal RA, Merkow RP, et al; American College of Surgeons National Surgical Quality Improvement Program; American Geriatrics Society: Optimal preoperative assessment of the geriatric surgical patient: a best practices guideline from the American College of Surgeons National Surgical Quality Improvement Program and the American Geriatrics Society. J Am Coll Surg 215(4):453–466, 2012 22917646
Chuen VL, Chan ACH, Ma J, et al: The frequency and quality of delirium documentation in discharge summaries. BMC Geriatr 21(1):307, 2021 33980170
Citrome L, Preskorn SH, Lauriello J, et al: Sublingual dexmedetomidine for the treatment of acute agitation in adults with schizophrenia or schizoaffective disorder: a randomized placebo-controlled trial. J Clin Psychiatry 83(6):22m14447, 2022
Code of Federal Regulations: Title 42, Chapter IV, Subchapter G, Part § 482.13: Condition of Participation: Patient's Rights. 2023. Available at: https://www.ecfr.gov/current/title-42/chapter-IV/subchapter-G/part-482. Accessed August 9, 2023.
Cole MG, McCusker J: Delirium in older adults: a chronic cognitive disorder? Int Psychogeriatr 28(8):1229–1233, 2016 27246118
Cole MG, McCusker J, Bailey R, et al: Partial and no recovery from delirium after hospital discharge predict increased adverse events. Age Ageing 46(1):90–95, 2017 28181649
Connell J, Oldham M, Pandharipande P, et al: Malignant catatonia: a review for the intensivist. J Intensive Care Med 38(2):137–150, 2023 35861966
Conteh E, Alorda A, Lebowitz D, et al: Disparities in the use of chemical and physical restraints in the emergency department by race/ethnicity. J Racial Ethn Health Disparities 11(1):132–136, 2024 36622570
Council of Medical Specialty Societies: Principles for the Development of Specialty Society Clinical Guidelines. Chicago, IL, Council of Medical Specialty Societies, 2017
Creamer M, Bell R, Failla S: Psychometric properties of the Impact of Event Scale - Revised. Behav Res Ther 41(12):1489–1496, 2003 14705607
Cui N, Yan X, Zhang Y, et al: Non-pharmacological interventions for minimizing physical restraints use in intensive care units: an umbrella review. Front Med (Lausanne) 9:806945, 2022 35573001
Cummings-Vaughn LA, Chavakula NN, Malmstrom TK, et al: Veterans Affairs Saint Louis University Mental Status examination compared with the Montreal Cognitive Assessment and the Short Test of Mental Status. J Am Geriatr Soc 62(7):1341–1346, 2014 24916485
Curry A, Malas N, Mroczkowski M, et al: Updates in the assessment and management of agitation. Focus (Am Psychiatr Publ) 21(1):35–45, 2023 37205032
Curtin D, Jennings E, Daunt R, et al: Deprescribing in older people approaching end of life: a randomized controlled trial using STOPPFrail criteria. J Am Geriatr Soc 68(4):762–769, 2020 31868920
D'Angelo RG, Rincavage M, Tata AL, et al: Impact of an antipsychotic discontinuation bundle during transitions of care in critically ill patients. J Intensive Care Med 34(1):40–47, 2019 28049388
Danish Health Authority: National Clinical Guideline for Prevention and Treatment of Organic Delirium: Quick Guide. Copenhagen, Danish Health Authority, May 2021. Available at: https://www.sst.dk/-/media/Udgivelser/2021/NKR-delirium/Eng-quick-guide_Forebyggelse-og-behandling-af-organisk-delirium.ashx. Accessed December 5, 2023.
Darwich AS, von Moltke L: The impact of formulation, delivery, and dosing regimen on the risk of drug-drug interactions. Clin Pharmacol Ther 105(6):1329–1331, 2019 30897206
De J, Wand AP: Delirium screening: a systematic review of delirium screening tools in hospitalized patients. Gerontologist 55(6):1079–1099, 2015 26543179
De Crescenzo F, D'Alò GL, Ostinelli EG, et al: Comparative effects of pharmacological interventions for the acute and long-term management of insomnia disorder in adults: a systematic review and network meta-analysis. Lancet 400(10347):170–184, 2022 35843245

de Lange E, Verhaak PF, van der Meer K: Prevalence, presentation and prognosis of delirium in older people in the population, at home and in long term care: a review. Int J Geriatr Psychiatry 28(2):127–134, 2013 22513757

Demeester C, Robins D, Edwina AE, et al: Physiologically based pharmacokinetic (PBPK) modelling of oral drug absorption in older adults - an AGePOP review. Eur J Pharm Sci 188:106496, 2023 37329924

de Negreiros DP, da Silva Meleiro AM, Furlanetto LM, et al: Portuguese version of the Delirium Rating Scale-Revised-98: reliability and validity. Int J Geriatr Psychiatry 23(5):472–477, 2008 17922493

Denysenko L, Sica N, Penders TM, et al; The Academy of Consultation-Liaison Psychiatry Evidence-Based Medicine Subcommittee Monograph: Catatonia in the medically ill: etiology, diagnosis, and treatment. Ann Clin Psychiatry 30(2):140–155, 2018 29697715

Derendorf H, Schmidt S: Rowland and Tozer's Clinical Pharmacokinetics and Pharmacodynamics: Concepts and Applications, 5th Edition. Philadelphia, PA, Wolters Kluwer, 2020

Devanand DP, Jeste DV, Stroup TS, et al: Overview of late-onset psychoses. Int Psychogeriatr 36(1):28–42, 2024 36866576

Devlin JW, Fong JJ, Schumaker G, et al: Use of a validated delirium assessment tool improves the ability of physicians to identify delirium in medical intensive care unit patients. Crit Care Med 35(12):2721–2724, quiz 2725, 2007 18074477

Devlin JW, Skrobik Y, Gélinas C, et al: Clinical practice guidelines for the prevention and management of pain, agitation/sedation, delirium, immobility, and sleep disruption in adult patients in the ICU. Crit Care Med 46(9):e825–e873, 2018 30113379

Dixit D, Barbarello Andrews L, Radparvar S, et al: Descriptive analysis of the unwarranted continuation of antipsychotics for the management of ICU delirium during transitions of care: a multicenter evaluation across New Jersey. Am J Health Syst Pharm 78(15):1385–1394, 2021 33895793

Djulbegovic B, Trikalinos TA, Roback J, et al: Impact of quality of evidence on the strength of recommendations: an empirical study. BMC Health Serv Res 9:120, 2009 19622148

Dosa D, Intrator O, McNicoll L, et al: Preliminary derivation of a nursing home confusion assessment method based on data from the minimum data set. J Am Geriatr Soc 55(7):1099–1105, 2007 17608886

Drewas L, Ghadir H, Neef R, et al: Individual Pharmacotherapy Management (IPM) - I: a group-matched retrospective controlled clinical study on prevention of complicating delirium in the elderly trauma patients and identification of associated factors. BMC Geriatr 22(1):29, 2022 34991474

Duceppe MA, Williamson DR, Elliott A, et al: Modifiable risk factors for delirium in critically ill trauma patients: a multicenter prospective study. J Intensive Care Med 34(4):330–336, 2019 28335673

Duggan MC, Van J, Ely EW: Delirium assessment in critically ill older adults: considerations during the COVID-19 pandemic. Crit Care Clin 37(1):175–190, 2021 33190768

Duong J, Wang G, Lean G, et al: Family-centered interventions and patient outcomes in the adult intensive care unit: a systematic review of randomized controlled trials. J Crit Care 83:154829, 2024 38759579

Duprey MS, van den Boogaard M, van der Hoeven JG, et al: Association between incident delirium and 28- and 90-day mortality in critically ill adults: a secondary analysis. Crit Care 24(1):161, 2020 32312288

Ely EW: Confusion Assessment Method for the ICU (CAM-ICU): The Complete Training Manual, Revised. Nashville, TN, Vanderbilt University, 2016. Available at: https://uploads-ssl.webflow.com/5b0849daec50243a0a1e5e0c/63c6c3d5e25c34cc55863461_The-Complete-CAM-ICU-training-manual-2016-08-31-3_Final.pdf. Accessed May 24, 2023.

Ely EW: The ABCDEF bundle: science and philosophy of how ICU liberation serves patients and families. Crit Care Med 45(2):321–330, 2017 28098628

Ely EW, Inouye SK, Bernard GR, et al: Delirium in mechanically ventilated patients: validity and reliability of the Confusion Assessment Method for the Intensive Care Unit (CAM-ICU). JAMA 286(21):2703–2710, 2001 11730446

Ely EW, Truman B, Shintani A, et al: Monitoring sedation status over time in ICU patients: reliability and validity of the Richmond Agitation-Sedation Scale (RASS). JAMA 289(22):2983–2991, 2003 12799407

Engstrom K, Mattson AE, Mara K, et al: Safety and effectiveness of benzodiazepines and antipsychotics for agitation in older adults in the emergency department. Am J Emerg Med 67:156–162, 2023 36893629

Erland LA, Saxena PK: Melatonin natural health products and supplements: presence of serotonin and significant variability of melatonin content. J Clin Sleep Med 13(2):275–281, 2017 27855744

Ertuğrul B, Özden D: The effect of physical restraint on neurovascular complications in intensive care units. Aust Crit Care 33(1):30–38, 2020 31079994

European Delirium Association, American Delirium Society: The DSM-5 criteria, level of arousal and delirium diagnosis: inclusiveness is safer. BMC Med 12:141, 2014 25300023

Evensen S, Hylen Ranhoff A, Lydersen S, et al: The delirium screening tool 4AT in routine clinical practice: prediction of mortality, sensitivity and specificity. Eur Geriatr Med 12(4):793–800, 2021 33813725

Featherstone I, Sheldon T, Johnson M, et al: Risk factors for delirium in adult patients receiving specialist palliative care: a systematic review and meta-analysis. Palliat Med 36(2):254–267, 2022 34930056

Fetters MB, Diep C, Ran R, et al: Effect of enteral guanfacine on dexmedetomidine use in the ICU. Crit Care Explor 4(11):e0785, 2022 36349291

Fick DM, Agostini JV, Inouye SK: Delirium superimposed on dementia: a systematic review. J Am Geriatr Soc 50(10):1723–1732, 2002 12366629

Fick DM, Jones RN, Inouye SK, et al: The Ultra-Brief Confusion Assessment Method (UB-CAM): A New Approach for Rapid Diagnosis of CAM-Defined Delirium. 2024. Available at: https://americandeliriumsociety.org/wp-content/uploads/2021/08/UB-CAM_Training-Manual.pdf. Accessed August 13, 2024.

Fiest KM, Soo A, Hee Lee C, et al: Long-term outcomes in ICU patients with delirium: a population-based cohort study. Am J Respir Crit Care Med 204(4):412–420, 2021 33823122

Finkelmeier F, Walter S, Peiffer KH, et al: Diagnostic yield and outcomes of computed tomography of the head in critically ill nontrauma patients. J Intensive Care Med 34(11-12):955–966, 2019 28718341
Flockhart DA, Thacker D, McDonald C, et al: The Flockhart Cytochrome P450 Drug-Drug Interaction Table. Bloomington, Division of Clinical Pharmacology, Indiana University School of Medicine, Updated 2021. Available at: https://drug-interactions.medicine.iu.edu. Accessed September 25, 2023.
Flurie RW, Gonzales JP, Tata AL, et al: Hospital delirium treatment: continuation of antipsychotic therapy from the intensive care unit to discharge. Am J Health Syst Pharm 72(23)(Suppl 3):S133–S139, 2015 26582298
Folstein MF, Folstein SE, McHugh PR: "Mini-mental state": a practical method for grading the cognitive state of patients for the clinician. J Psychiatr Res 12(3):189–198, 1975 1202204
Folstein MF, Folstein SE, Messer MA, et al: Mini-Mental State Examination, 2nd Edition (MMSE-2). Lutz, FL, Psychological Assessment Resources, 2010
Fong TG, Inouye SK: The inter-relationship between delirium and dementia: the importance of delirium prevention. Nat Rev Neurol 18(10):579–596, 2022 36028563
Fong TG, Davis D, Growdon ME, et al: The interface between delirium and dementia in elderly adults. Lancet Neurol 14(8):823–832, 2015 26139023
Fong TG, Racine AM, Fick DM, et al: The caregiver burden of delirium in older adults with Alzheimer disease and related disorders. J Am Geriatr Soc 67(12):2587–2592, 2019 31605539
Fong TG, Hshieh TT, Tabloski PA, et al: Identifying delirium in persons with moderate or severe dementia: review of challenges and an illustrative approach. Am J Geriatr Psychiatry 30(10):1067–1078, 2022 35581117
Franco JG, Mejía MA, Ochoa SB, et al: Delirium Rating Scale-Revised-98 (DRS-R-98): Colombian adaptation of the Spanish version [in Spanish]. Actas Esp Psiquiatr 35(3):170–175, 2007 17508293
Franco JG, Trzepacz PT, Meagher DJ, et al: Three core domains of delirium validated using exploratory and confirmatory factor analyses. Psychosomatics 54(3):227–238, 2013 23218057
Franco JG, Ocampo MV, Velásquez-Tirado JD, et al: Validation of the Delirium Diagnostic Tool-Provisional (DDT-Pro) with medical inpatients and comparison with the Confusion Assessment Method algorithm. J Neuropsychiatry Clin Neurosci 32(3):213–226, 2020a 31662094
Franco JG, Trzepacz PT, Sepúlveda E, et al: Delirium Diagnostic Tool-Provisional (DDT-Pro) scores in delirium, subsyndromal delirium and no delirium. Gen Hosp Psychiatry 67:107–114, 2020b 33091783
Franks ZM, Alcock JA, Lam T, et al: Physical restraints and post-traumatic stress disorder in survivors of critical illness: a systematic review and meta-analysis. Ann Am Thorac Soc 18(4):689–697, 2021 33075240
Friberg K, Hofsø K, Ræder J, et al: Prevalence of and predictive factors associated with high levels of post-traumatic stress symptoms 3 months after intensive care unit admission: a prospective study. Aust Crit Care 37(2):222–229, 2024 37455211
Fried LP, Cohen AA, Xue QL, et al: The physical frailty syndrome as a transition from homeostatic symphony to cacophony. Nat Aging 1(1):36–46, 2021 34476409
Funayama M, Takata T: Psychiatric inpatients subjected to physical restraint have a higher risk of deep vein thrombosis and aspiration pneumonia. Gen Hosp Psychiatry 62:1–5, 2020 31734627
Funk MC, Beach SR, Bostwick JR, et al: Resource Document on QTc Prolongation and Psychotropic Medications. APA Resource Document. Washington, DC, American Psychiatric Association, 2018. Available at: https://www.psychiatry.org/File%20Library/Psychiatrists/Directories/Library-and-Archive/resource_documents/Resource-Document-2018-QTc-Prolongation-and-Psychotropic-Med.pdf. Accessed October 10, 2023.
Furlan AD, Malmivaara A, Chou R, et al; Editorial Board of the Cochrane Back, Neck Group: 2015 updated method guideline for systematic reviews in the Cochrane Back and Neck Group. Spine 40(21):1660–1673, 2015 26208232
Gaete Ortega D, Papathanassoglou E, Norris CM: The lived experience of delirium in intensive care unit patients: a meta-ethnography. Aust Crit Care 33(2):193–202, 2020 30871853
Gage L, Hogan DB: 2014 Guideline Update: The Assessment and Treatment of Delirium. Toronto, ON, Canadian Coalition for Seniors' Mental Health, 2014. Available at: https://ccsmh.ca/wp-content/uploads/2016/03/2014-ccsmh-Guideline-Update-Delirium.pdf. Accessed December 5, 2023.
Galvin JE, Roe CM, Powlishta KK, et al: The AD8: a brief informant interview to detect dementia. Neurology 65(4):559–564, 2005 16116116
Gaudreau JD, Gagnon P, Harel F, et al: Fast, systematic, and continuous delirium assessment in hospitalized patients: the nursing delirium screening scale. J Pain Symptom Manage 29(4):368–375, 2005 15857740
Gélinas C, Bérubé M, Chevrier A, et al: Delirium assessment tools for use in critically ill adults: a psychometric analysis and systematic review. Crit Care Nurse 38(1):38–49, 2018 29437077
Geodon (ziprasidone) [prescribing information]. New York, Pfizer Inc, February 2022
Geriatric Medicine Research Collaborative: Delirium is prevalent in older hospital inpatients and associated with adverse outcomes: results of a prospective multi-centre study on World Delirium Awareness Day. BMC Med 17(1):229, 2019 31837711
Gessner A, König J, Fromm MF: Clinical aspects of transporter-mediated drug-drug interactions. Clin Pharmacol Ther 105(6):1386–1394, 2019 30648735
Ghezzi ES, Greaves D, Boord MS, et al: How do predisposing factors differ between delirium motor subtypes? A systematic review and meta-analysis. Age Ageing 51(9):afac200, 2022 36153750
Gibb K, Seeley A, Quinn T, et al: The consistent burden in published estimates of delirium occurrence in medical inpatients over four decades: a systematic review and meta-analysis study. Age Ageing 49(3):352–360, 2020 32239173
Giedzinska A, Wilson AR: The Clinician's Handbook on Measurement-Based Care: The How, the What, and the Why Bother. Washington, DC, American Psychiatric Association Publishing, 2023

Girard TD, Exline MC, Carson SS, et al; MIND-USA Investigators: Haloperidol and ziprasidone for treatment of delirium in critical illness. N Engl J Med 379(26):2506–2516, 2018 30346242

Glaess SS, Attridge RL, Christina Gutierrez G: Clonidine as a strategy for discontinuing dexmedetomidine sedation in critically ill patients: a narrative review. Am J Health Syst Pharm 77(7):515–522, 2020 32086509

Goldberg TE, Chen C, Wang Y, et al: Association of delirium with long-term cognitive decline: a meta-analysis. JAMA Neurol 77(11):1373–1381, 2020 32658246

Gonzalez J, Upadhyaya VD, Manna ZT, et al: Paradoxical excitation following intravenous lorazepam administration for alcohol withdrawal - a case presentation and literature review. J Pharm Pract 36(5):1244–1248, 2023 35466771

Gou RY, Hshieh TT, Marcantonio ER, et al; SAGES Study Group: One-year Medicare costs associated with delirium in older patients undergoing major elective surgery. JAMA Surg 156(5):430–442, 2021 33625501

Gouju J, Legeay S: Pharmacokinetics of obese adults: not only an increase in weight. Biomed Pharmacother 166:115281, 2023 37573660

Grassi L, Caruso R, Da Ronch C, et al: Quality of life, level of functioning, and its relationship with mental and physical disorders in the elderly: results from the MentDis_ICF65+ study. Health Qual Life Outcomes 18(1):61, 2020 32143635

Greaves D, Psaltis PJ, Davis DHJ, et al: Risk factors for delirium and cognitive decline following coronary artery bypass grafting surgery: a systematic review and meta-analysis. J Am Heart Assoc 9(22):e017275, 2020 33164631

Greenwald JL, Halasyamani L, Greene J, et al: Making inpatient medication reconciliation patient centered, clinically relevant and implementable: a consensus statement on key principles and necessary first steps. J Hosp Med 5(8):477–485, 2010 20945473

Griffin TT, Bhave V, McNulty J, et al: Delirium and previous psychiatric history independently predict poststroke posttraumatic stress disorder. Neurologist 28(6):362–366, 2023 37083500

Grossmann FF, Hasemann W, Graber A, et al: Screening, detection and management of delirium in the emergency department - a pilot study on the feasibility of a new algorithm for use in older emergency department patients: the modified Confusion Assessment Method for the Emergency Department (mCAM-ED). Scand J Trauma Resusc Emerg Med 22:19, 2014 24625212

Grover S, Kate N: Assessment scales for delirium: a review. World J Psychiatry 2(4):58–70, 2012 24175169

Guinart D, Misawa F, Rubio JM, et al: A systematic review and pooled, patient-level analysis of predictors of mortality in neuroleptic malignant syndrome. Acta Psychiatr Scand 144(4):329–341, 2021 34358327

Guthrie PF, Rayborn S, Butcher HK: Evidence-based practice guideline: delirium. J Gerontol Nurs 44(2):14–24, 2018 29378075

Guyatt G, Gutterman D, Baumann MH, et al: Grading strength of recommendations and quality of evidence in clinical guidelines: report from an American College of Chest Physicians task force. Chest 129(1):174–181, 2006 16424429

Guyatt GH, Oxman AD, Kunz R, et al; GRADE Working Group: Going from evidence to recommendations. BMJ 336(7652):1049–1051, 2008 18467413

Guyatt G, Eikelboom JW, Akl EA, et al: A guide to GRADE guidelines for the readers of JTH. J Thromb Haemost 11(8):1603–1608, 2013 23773710

Haimovich AD, Taylor RA, Chang-Sing E, et al: Disparities associated with electronic behavioral alerts for safety and violence concerns in the emergency department. Ann Emerg Med 83(2):100–107, 2024 37269262

Haldol lactate injection (haloperidol) [prescribing information]. Titusville, NJ, Janssen Pharmaceuticals Inc, November 2020

Haley MN, Casey P, Kane RY, et al: Delirium management: let's get physical? A systematic review and meta-analysis. Australas J Ageing 38(4):231–241, 2019 30793460

Halladay CW, Sillner AY, Rudolph JL: Performance of electronic prediction rules for prevalent delirium at hospital admission. JAMA Netw Open 1(4):e181405, 2018 30646122

Haloperidol [prescribing information]. Princeton, NJ, Sandoz, Inc, September 2008

Haloperidol [product monograph]. Caledon, ON, Canada, Neo Health Canada, Inc, November 2019

Haloperidol lactate [prescribing information]. Greenville, SC, Pharmaceutical Associates, Inc, December 2008

Haloperidol lactate injection [prescribing information]. Schaumburg, IL, Sagent Pharmaceuticals, August 2011

Haloperidol lactate oral solution [prescribing information]. Greenville, SC, Pharmaceutical Associates, Inc, November 2016

Haloperidol lactate oral solution USP (concentrate) [prescribing information]. Greenville, SC, Pharmaceutical Associates, Inc, March 2020

Haloperidol tablets [prescribing information]. Princeton, NJ, Sandoz, Inc, July 2015

Haloperidol tablets [prescribing information]. Maple Grove, MN, Upsher-Smith Laboratories, LLC, June 2019

Han JH: Brief Confusion Assessment Method (bCAM) Instruction Manual v1, October 15, 2015. Nashville, TN, Vanderbilt University, 2015. Available at: https://eddelirium.org/wp-content/uploads/2016/05/bCAM-Training-Manual-Version-1.0-10-15-2015.pdf. Accessed July 20, 2024.

Han JH, Wilson A, Vasilevskis EE, et al: Diagnosing delirium in older emergency department patients: validity and reliability of the delirium triage screen and the brief Confusion Assessment Method. Ann Emerg Med 62(5):457–465, 2013 23916018

Han QYC, Rodrigues NG, Klainin-Yobas P, et al: Prevalence, risk factors, and impact of delirium on hospitalized older adults with dementia: a systematic review and meta-analysis. J Am Med Dir Assoc 23(1):23–32.e27, 2022 34648761

Harris J, Ramelet AS, van Dijk M, et al: Clinical recommendations for pain, sedation, withdrawal and delirium assessment in critically ill infants and children: an ESPNIC position statement for healthcare professionals. Intensive Care Med 42(6):972–986, 2016 27084344

Harris RP, Helfand M, Woolf SH, et al; Methods Work Group, Third U.S. Preventive Services Task Force: Current methods of the US Preventive Services Task Force: a review of the process. Am J Prev Med 20(3 Suppl):21–35, 2001 11306229

Hassan S, Hasnain Z, Awan K, et al: Effect of peri-operative dexmedetomidine on incidence of delirium in elderly patients after cardiac surgery. Med Forum 32(2):142–146, 2021

Hasuo H, Kanbara K, Fujii R, et al: Factors associated with the effectiveness of intravenous administration of chlorpromazine for delirium in patients with terminal cancer. J Palliat Med 21(9):1257–1264, 2018 29757064

Hatchett C, Langley G, Schmollgruber S: Psychological sequelae following ICU admission at a level 1 academic South African hospital. South Afr J Crit Care 26:52–58, 2010

Hawkins M, Sockalingam S, Bonato S, et al: A rapid review of the pathoetiology, presentation, and management of delirium in adults with COVID-19. J Psychosom Res 141:110350, 2021 33401078

Hazlehurst JM, Armstrong MJ, Sherlock M, et al: A comparative quality assessment of evidence-based clinical guidelines in endocrinology. Clin Endocrinol (Oxf) 78(2):183–190, 2013 22624723

He F, Shen L, Zhong J: A study of dexmedetomidine in the prevention of postoperative delirium in elderly patients after vertebral osteotomy. Int J Clin Exp Med 11(5):4984–4990, 2018

Heavner MS, Louzon PR, Gorman EF, et al: A rapid systematic review of pharmacologic sleep promotion modalities in the intensive care unit. J Intensive Care Med 39(1):28–43, 2024 37403460

Helfand BKI, D'Aquila ML, Tabloski P, et al: Detecting delirium: a systematic review of identification instruments for non-ICU settings. J Am Geriatr Soc 69(2):547–555, 2021 33135780

Hendset M, Haslemo T, Rudberg I, et al: The complexity of active metabolites in therapeutic drug monitoring of psychotropic drugs. Pharmacopsychiatry 39(4):121–127, 2006 16871467

Herzig SJ, LaSalvia MT, Naidus E, et al: Antipsychotics and the risk of aspiration pneumonia in individuals hospitalized for nonpsychiatric conditions: a cohort study. J Am Geriatr Soc 65(12):2580–2586, 2017 29095482

Higgins JPT, Savović J, Page MJ, et al: Risk of bias in randomized trials, in Cochrane Handbook for Systematic Reviews of Interventions, Version 6.4. Edited by Higgins JPT, Thomas J, Chandler J, et al. London, Cochrane, 2023. Available at: www.training.cochrane.org/handbook. Accessed December 11, 2023.

Hospira: Droperidol. Lake Forest, IL, Hospira, Inc, 2021. Available at: https://americanregent.com/media/1574/droperidol_prescribing-information.pdf. Accessed April 6, 2025.

Hospira: Precedex- Dexmedetomidine Hydrochloride Injection, Solution [prescribing information]. Lake Forest, IL, Hospira, Inc, November 2023. Available at: https://labeling.pfizer.com/ShowLabeling.aspx?id=4404. Accessed April 27, 2024.

Hshieh TT, Yang T, Gartaganis SL, et al: Hospital Elder Life Program: systematic review and meta-analysis of effectiveness. Am J Geriatr Psychiatry 26(10):1015–1033, 2018 30076080

Hshieh TT, Inouye SK, Oh ES: Delirium in the elderly. Clin Geriatr Med 36(2):183–199, 2020 32222295

Huang MC, Lee CH, Lai YC, et al: Chinese version of the Delirium Rating Scale-Revised-98: reliability and validity. Compr Psychiatry 50(1):81–85, 2009 19059519

Huang Q, Xie Y, Hu Z, et al: Anti-N-methyl-D-aspartate receptor encephalitis: a review of pathogenic mechanisms, treatment, prognosis. Brain Res 1727:146549, 2020 31726044

Hughes CG, Hayhurst CJ, Pandharipande PP, et al: Association of delirium during critical illness with mortality: multicenter prospective cohort study. Anesth Analg 133(5):1152–1161, 2021 33929361

Hui D, De La Rosa A, Wilson A, et al: Neuroleptic strategies for terminal agitation in patients with cancer and delirium at an acute palliative care unit: a single-centre, double-blind, parallel-group, randomised trial. Lancet Oncol 21(7):989–998, 2020 32479786

Hunt NF, McLaughlin KC, Kovacevic MP, et al: Safety of intravenous olanzapine administration at a tertiary academic medical center. Ann Pharmacother 55(9):1127–1133, 2021 33455436

Iamaroon A, Wongviriyawong T, Sura-Arunsumrit P, et al: Incidence of and risk factors for postoperative delirium in older adult patients undergoing noncardiac surgery: a prospective study. BMC Geriatr 20(1):40, 2020 32013872

Inouye SK: The Short Confusion Assessment Method (Short CAM): Training Manual and Coding Guide. Boston, MA, Hospital Elder Life Program, 2014. Available at: https://americandeliriumsociety.org/wp-content/uploads/2021/08/CAM-S_TrainingManual.pdf. Accessed April 7, 2025.

Inouye SK: The importance of delirium and delirium prevention in older adults during lockdowns. JAMA 325(17):1779–1780, 2021 33720288

Inouye SK, van Dyck CH, Alessi CA, et al: Clarifying confusion: the confusion assessment method. A new method for detection of delirium. Ann Intern Med 113(12):941–948, 1990 2240918

Inouye SK, Bogardus ST Jr, Baker DI, et al; Hospital Elder Life Program: The Hospital Elder Life Program: a model of care to prevent cognitive and functional decline in older hospitalized patients. J Am Geriatr Soc 48(12):1697–1706, 2000 11129764

Inouye SK, Foreman MD, Mion LC, et al: Nurses' recognition of delirium and its symptoms: comparison of nurse and researcher ratings. Arch Intern Med 161(20):2467–2473, 2001 11700159

Inouye SK, Bogardus ST Jr, Williams CS, et al: The role of adherence on the effectiveness of nonpharmacologic interventions: evidence from the delirium prevention trial. Arch Intern Med 163(8):958–964, 2003 12719206

Inouye SK, Marcantonio ER, Kosar CM, et al: The short-term and long-term relationship between delirium and cognitive trajectory in older surgical patients. Alzheimers Dement 12(7):766–775, 2016 27103261

Institute of Medicine: Clinical Practice Guidelines We Can Trust. Washington, DC, National Academies Press, 2011

Israni J, Lesser A, Kent T, et al: Delirium as a predictor of mortality in US Medicare beneficiaries discharged from the emergency department: a national claims-level analysis up to 12 months. BMJ Open 8(5):e021258, 2018 29730630

Ista E, Traube C, de Neef M, et al; Dutch Multidisciplinary Pediatric Delirium Guideline Group: Factors associated with delirium in children: a systematic review and meta-analysis. Pediatr Crit Care Med 24(5):372–381, 2023 36790201

Jaimes-Albornoz W, Ruiz de Pellon-Santamaria A, Nizama-Vía A, et al: Catatonia in older adults: a systematic review. World J Psychiatry 12(2):348–367, 2022 35317341

Jakob SM, Ruokonen E, Grounds RM, et al; Dexmedetomidine for Long-Term Sedation Investigators: Dexmedetomidine vs midazolam or propofol for sedation during prolonged mechanical ventilation: two randomized controlled trials. JAMA 307(11):1151–1160, 2012 22436955

Jaworska N, Moss SJ, Krewulak KD, et al: A scoping review of perceptions from healthcare professionals on antipsychotic prescribing practices in acute care settings. BMC Health Serv Res 22(1):1272, 2022 36271347

Jin Z, Hu J, Ma D: Postoperative delirium: perioperative assessment, risk reduction, and management. Br J Anaesth 125(4):492–504, 2020 32798069

Johnson KG, Fashoyin A, Madden-Fuentes R, et al: Discharge plans for geriatric inpatients with delirium: a plan to stop antipsychotics? J Am Geriatr Soc 65(10):2278–2281, 2017 28856665

Johnson TJ, Hickey RW, Switzer GE, et al: The impact of cognitive stressors in the emergency department on physician implicit racial bias. Acad Emerg Med 23(3):297–305, 2016 26763939

Johnston KJ, Chin MH, Pollack HA: Health equity for individuals with intellectual and developmental disabilities. JAMA 328(16):1587–1588, 2022 36206010

Jones C, Bäckman C, Capuzzo M, et al: Precipitants of post-traumatic stress disorder following intensive care: a hypothesis generating study of diversity in care. Intensive Care Med 33(6):978–985, 2007 17384929

Jorm AF: A short form of the Informant Questionnaire on Cognitive Decline in the Elderly (IQCODE): development and cross-validation. Psychol Med 24(1):145–153, 1994 8208879

Jorm AF, Jacomb PA: The Informant Questionnaire on Cognitive Decline in the Elderly (IQCODE): socio-demographic correlates, reliability, validity and some norms. Psychol Med 19(4):1015–1022, 1989 2594878

Kang SY, Seo SW, Kim JY: Comprehensive risk factor evaluation of postoperative delirium following major surgery: clinical data warehouse analysis. Neurol Sci 40(4):793–800, 2019 30675675

Kato M, Kishi Y, Okuyama T, et al: Japanese version of the Delirium Rating Scale, Revised-98 (DRS-R98-J): reliability and validity. Psychosomatics 51(5):425–431, 2010 20833942

Kean J, Trzepacz PT, Murray LL, et al: Initial validation of a brief provisional diagnostic scale for delirium. Brain Inj 24(10):1222–1230, 2010 20645705

Keating GM: Dexmedetomidine: a review of its use for sedation in the intensive care setting. Drugs 75(10):1119–1130, 2015 26063213

Keller F, Hann A: Clinical pharmacodynamics: principles of drug response and alterations in kidney disease. Clin J Am Soc Nephrol 13(9):1413–1420, 2018 29769182

Khan BA, Perkins AJ, Gao S, et al: The Confusion Assessment Method for the ICU-7 delirium severity scale: a novel delirium severity instrument for use in the ICU. Crit Care Med 45(5):851–857, 2017 28263192

Khatri UG, Delgado MK, South E, et al: Racial disparities in the management of emergency department patients presenting with psychiatric disorders. Ann Epidemiol 69:9–16, 2022 35227925

Kiang TK, Ensom MH, Chang TK: UDP-glucuronosyltransferases and clinical drug-drug interactions. Pharmacol Ther 106(1):97–132, 2005 15781124

Killin L, Hezam A, Anderson KK, et al: Advanced medication reconciliation: a systematic review of the impact on medication errors and adverse drug events associated with transitions of care. Jt Comm J Qual Patient Saf 47(7):438–451, 2021 34103267

Kim K, Jeong JH, Choi EK: Non-pharmacological interventions for delirium in the pediatric population: a systematic review with narrative synthesis. BMC Pediatr 24(1):108, 2024 38347509

Kinchin I, Mitchell E, Agar M, et al: The economic cost of delirium: a systematic review and quality assessment. Alzheimers Dement 17(6):1026–1041, 2021 33480183

King AJ, Potter KM, Seaman JB, et al: Measuring performance on the ABCDEF bundle during interprofessional rounds via a nurse-based assessment tool. Am J Crit Care 32(2):92–99, 2023 36854912

Klein Klouwenberg PM, Zaal IJ, Spitoni C, et al: The attributable mortality of delirium in critically ill patients: prospective cohort study. BMJ 349:g6652, 2014 25422275

Knauert MP, Ayas NT, Bosma KJ, et al: Causes, consequences, and treatments of sleep and circadian disruption in the ICU: an official American Thoracic Society research statement. Am J Respir Crit Care Med 207(7):e49–e68, 2023 36999950

Knox DK, Holloman GH Jr: Use and avoidance of seclusion and restraint: consensus statement of the American Association for Emergency Psychiatry Project Beta Seclusion and Restraint Workgroup. West J Emerg Med 13(1):35–40, 2012 22461919

Korczak V, Kirby A, Gunja N: Chemical agents for the sedation of agitated patients in the ED: a systematic review. Am J Emerg Med 34(12):2426–2431, 2016 27707527

Kotfis K, Marra A, Ely EW: ICU delirium - a diagnostic and therapeutic challenge in the intensive care unit. Anaesthesiol Intensive Ther 50(2):160–167, 2018 29882581

Kotfis K, Williams Roberson S, Wilson J, et al: COVID-19: what do we need to know about ICU delirium during the SARS-CoV-2 pandemic? Anaesthesiol Intensive Ther 52(2):132–138, 2020 32419438

Kram BL, Schultheis JM, Kram SJ, et al: A pharmacy-based electronic handoff tool to reduce discharge prescribing of atypical antipsychotics initiated in the intensive care unit: a quality improvement initiative. J Pharm Pract 32(4):434–441, 2019 29486664

Krewulak KD, Stelfox HT, Leigh JP, et al: Incidence and prevalence of delirium subtypes in an adult ICU: a systematic review and meta-analysis. Crit Care Med 46(12):2029–2035, 2018 30234569

Krewulak KD, Stelfox HT, Ely EW, et al: Risk factors and outcomes among delirium subtypes in adult ICUs: a systematic review. J Crit Care 56:257–264, 2020 31986369

Krinitski D, Kasina R, Klöppel S, et al: Associations of delirium with urinary tract infections and asymptomatic bacteriuria in adults aged 65 and older: a systematic review and meta-analysis. J Am Geriatr Soc 69(11):3312–3323, 2021 34448496

Kroenke K, Spitzer RL, Williams JB: The PHQ-9: validity of a brief depression severity measure. J Gen Intern Med 16(9):606–613, 2001 11556941

Krüger BD, Kurmann J, Corti N, et al: Dexmedetomidine-associated hyperthermia: a series of 9 cases and a review of the literature. Anesth Analg 125(6):1898–1906, 2017 28763361

Kukreja D, Günther U, Popp J: Delirium in the elderly: current problems with increasing geriatric age. Indian J Med Res 142(6):655–662, 2015 26831414

Kunicki ZJ, Ngo LH, Marcantonio ER, et al: Six-year cognitive trajectory in older adults following major surgery and delirium. JAMA Intern Med 183(5):442–450, 2023 36939716

Lagu T, Haywood C, Reimold K, et al: 'I am not the doctor for you': physicians' attitudes about caring for people with disabilities. Health Aff (Millwood) 41(10):1387–1395, 2022 36190896

Lai JY, Kalk N, Roberts E: The effectiveness and tolerability of anti-seizure medication in alcohol withdrawal syndrome: a systematic review, meta-analysis and GRADE of the evidence. Addiction 117(1):5–18, 2022 33822427

Lambert J, Vermassen J, Fierens J, et al: Discharge from hospital with newly administered antipsychotics after intensive care unit delirium - incidence and contributing factors. J Crit Care 61:162–167, 2021 33171333

Lange S, Mędrzycka-Dąbrowska W, Friganović A, et al: Family experiences and attitudes toward care of ICU patients with delirium: a scoping review. Front Public Health 10:1060518, 2022 36505003

Lee J, Negm A, Peters R, et al: Deprescribing fall-risk increasing drugs (FRIDs) for the prevention of falls and fall-related complications: a systematic review and meta-analysis. BMJ Open 11(2):e035978, 2021 33568364

Lee JS, Tong T, Chignell M, et al: Prevalence, management and outcomes of unrecognized delirium in a national sample of 1,493 older emergency department patients: how many were sent home and what happened to them? Age Ageing 51(2):afab214, 2022 35150585

Lee J, Yeom I, Yoo S, et al: Educational intervention for family caregivers of older adults with delirium: an integrative review. J Clin Nurs 32(19-20):6987–6997, 2023 37370251

Lee S, Cavalier FR, Hayes JM, et al: Delirium, confusion, or altered mental status as a risk for abnormal head CT in older adults in the emergency department: a systematic review and meta-analysis. Am J Emerg Med 71:190–194, 2023 37423026

Lee Y, Ryu J, Lee J, et al: Korean version of the Delirium Rating Scale-Revised-98: reliability and validity. Psychiatry Investig 8(1):30–38, 2011 21519534

Lee-Steere K, Mudge A, Liddle J, et al: Understanding family carer experiences and perceptions of engagement in delirium prevention and care for adults in hospital: qualitative systematic review. J Clin Nurs 33(4):1320–1345, 2024 38284503

Leonard M, Godfrey A, Silberhorn M, et al: Motion analysis in delirium: a novel method of clarifying motoric subtypes. Neurocase 13(4):272–277, 2007 17943614

Leonard M, Adamis D, Saunders J, et al: A longitudinal study of delirium phenomenology indicates widespread neural dysfunction. Palliat Support Care 13(2):187–196, 2015 24183238

Leslie DL, Marcantonio ER, Zhang Y, et al: One-year health care costs associated with delirium in the elderly population. Arch Intern Med 168(1):27–32, 2008 18195192

Levenson JL, Ferrando SJ (eds): Clinical Manual of Psychopharmacology in the Medically Ill, 3rd Edition. Washington, DC, American Psychiatric Association Publishing, 2024

Lewis K, Alshamsi F, Carayannopoulos KL, et al; GUIDE group: Dexmedetomidine vs other sedatives in critically ill mechanically ventilated adults: a systematic review and meta-analysis of randomized trials. Intensive Care Med 48(7):811–840, 2022 35648198

Lexi-Drugs: UpToDate Lexidrug. Waltham, MA, UpToDate, Inc, 2024. Available at: https://www.wolterskluwer.com/en/solutions/uptodate/pro/lexidrug. Accessed August 16, 2024.

Li HC, Yeh TY, Wei YC, et al: Association of incident delirium with short-term mortality in adults with critical illness receiving mechanical ventilation. JAMA Netw Open 5(10):e2235339, 2022 36205994

Li HC, Chen CC, Yeh TY, et al: Predicting hospital mortality and length of stay: a prospective cohort study comparing the Intensive Care Delirium Screening Checklist versus Confusion Assessment Method for the Intensive Care Unit. Aust Crit Care 36(3):378–384, 2023 35272910

Lin CJ, Su IC, Huang SW, et al: Delirium assessment tools among hospitalized older adults: a systematic review and metaanalysis of diagnostic accuracy. Ageing Res Rev 90:102025, 2023 37527704

Linnet K, Ejsing TB: A review on the impact of P-glycoprotein on the penetration of drugs into the brain: focus on psychotropic drugs. Eur Neuropsychopharmacol 18(3):157–169, 2008 17683917

Liu SW, Lee S, Hayes JM, et al; Geriatric Emergency Department Delirium Guidelines Group: Head computed tomography findings in geriatric emergency department patients with delirium, altered mental status, and confusion: a systematic review. Acad Emerg Med 30(6):616–625, 2023 36330667

Luccarelli J, Sacks CA, Snydeman C, et al: Coding for physical restraint status among hospitalized patients: a 2019 National Inpatient Sample Analysis. J Gen Intern Med 38(11):2461–2469, 2023 37002459

Ma R, Zhao J, Li C, et al: Diagnostic accuracy of the 3-minute diagnostic interview for confusion assessment method-defined delirium in delirium detection: a systematic review and meta-analysis. Age Ageing 52(5):afad074, 2023 37211364

MacLullich AMJ: 4AT: Rapid Clinical Test for Delirium website. 2024. Available at: https://www.the4at.com. Accessed January 10, 2024.

MacLullich AMJ, Hosie A, Tieges Z, et al: Three key areas in progressing delirium practice and knowledge: recognition and relief of distress, new directions in delirium epidemiology and developing better research assessments. Age Ageing 51(11):afac271, 2022 36441120

Maldonado JR: Acute brain failure: pathophysiology, diagnosis, management, and sequelae of delirium. Crit Care Clin 33(3):461–519, 2017 28601132

Maldonado JR, Wysong A, van der Starre PJ, et al: Dexmedetomidine and the reduction of postoperative delirium after cardiac surgery. Psychosomatics 50(3):206–217, 2009 19567759

Mancuso CE, Tanzi MG, Gabay M: Paradoxical reactions to benzodiazepines: literature review and treatment options. Pharmacotherapy 24(9):1177–1185, 2004 15460178

Mangoni AA, Jackson SH: Age-related changes in pharmacokinetics and pharmacodynamics: basic principles and practical applications. Br J Clin Pharmacol 57(1):6–14, 2004 14678335

Marcantonio ER: Delirium in hospitalized older adults. N Engl J Med 377(15):1456–1466, 2017 29020579

Marcantonio ER, Ngo LH, O'Connor M, et al: 3D-CAM: derivation and validation of a 3-minute diagnostic interview for CAM-defined delirium: a cross-sectional diagnostic test study. Ann Intern Med 161(8):554–561, 2014 25329203

Marcantonio ER, Fick DM, Jones RN, et al: The Ultra-Brief Confusion Assessment Method (UB-CAM): a new approach for rapid diagnosis of CAM-defined delirium. Network for Investigation of Delirium: Unifying Scientists (NIDUS). Boston, MA, July 2020. Available at: https://deliriumnetwork.org/the-ultra-brief-confusion-assessment-method-ub-cam. Accessed August 13, 2024.

Marcantonio ER, Fick DM, Jung Y, et al: Comparative implementation of a brief app-directed protocol for delirium identification by hospitalists, nurses, and nursing assistants: a cohort study. Ann Intern Med 175(1):65–73, 2022 34748377

Markota M, Rummans TA, Bostwick JM, et al: Benzodiazepine use in older adults: dangers, management, and alternative therapies. Mayo Clin Proc 91(11):1632–1639, 2016 27814838

Marquetand J, Bode L, Fuchs S, et al: Risk factors for delirium are different in the very old: a comparative one-year prospective cohort study of 5,831 patients. Front Psychiatry 12:655087, 2021 34045981

Marquetand J, Gehrke S, Bode L, et al: Delirium in trauma patients: a 1-year prospective cohort study of 2026 patients. Eur J Trauma Emerg Surg 48(2):1017–1024, 2022 33538844

Marra A, Ely EW, Pandharipande PP, et al: The ABCDEF bundle in critical care. Crit Care Clin 33(2):225–243, 2017 28284292

Marshall J, Hayes BD, Koehl J, et al: Effects of a pharmacy-driven medication history program on patient outcomes. Am J Health Syst Pharm 79(19):1652–1662, 2022 35596269

Mart MF, Williams Roberson S, Salas B, et al: Prevention and management of delirium in the intensive care unit. Semin Respir Crit Care Med 42(1):112–126, 2021 32746469

Martel ML, Klein LR, Rivard RL, et al: A large retrospective cohort of patients receiving intravenous olanzapine in the emergency department. Acad Emerg Med 23(1):29–35, 2016 26720055

Martin J, Heymann A, Bäsell K, et al: Evidence and consensus-based German guidelines for the management of analgesia, sedation and delirium in intensive care--short version. Ger Med Sci 8:Doc02, 2010 20200655

Maruani J, Reynaud E, Chambe J, et al: Efficacy of melatonin and ramelteon for the acute and long-term management of insomnia disorder in adults: a systematic review and meta-analysis. J Sleep Res 32(6):e13939, 2023 37434463

Matsuura Y, Ohno Y, Toyoshima M, et al: Effects of non-pharmacologic prevention on delirium in critically ill patients: a network meta-analysis. Nurs Crit Care 28(5):727–737, 2023 35624556

Mattison MLP: Delirium. Ann Intern Med 173(7):ITC49–ITC64, 2020 33017552

Mauri V, Reuter K, Körber MI, et al: Incidence, risk factors and impact on long-term outcome of postoperative delirium after transcatheter aortic valve replacement. Front Cardiovasc Med 8:645724, 2021 33842564

Maust DT, Kim HM, Seyfried LS, et al: Antipsychotics, other psychotropics, and the risk of death in patients with dementia: number needed to harm. JAMA Psychiatry 72(5):438–445, 2015 25786075

McCartney H, Noble E, MacLullich AMJ, et al: A systematic review of studies reporting on neuropsychological and functional domains used for assessment of recovery from delirium in acute hospital patients. Int J Geriatr Psychiatry 38(6):e5943, 2023 37294207

McDonald EG, Wu PE, Rashidi B, et al: The MedSafer study-electronic decision support for deprescribing in hospitalized older adults: a cluster randomized clinical trial. JAMA Intern Med 182(3):265–273, 2022 35040926

McKenzie J, Joy A: Family intervention improves outcomes for patients with delirium: systematic review and meta-analysis. Australas J Ageing 39(1):21–30, 2020 31250961

Meagher D, Leonard M: The active management of delirium: improving detection and treatment. Adv Psychiatr Treat 14(4):292–301, 2008

Meagher D, Moran M, Raju B, et al: A new data-based motor subtype schema for delirium. J Neuropsychiatry Clin Neurosci 20(2):185–193, 2008 18451189

Meagher D, O'Regan N, Ryan D, et al: Frequency of delirium and subsyndromal delirium in an adult acute hospital population. Br J Psychiatry 205(6):478–485, 2014 25359923

Megna BW, Vaughn BP: Therapeutic drug monitoring in practice for inflammatory bowel disease. Curr Gastroenterol Rep 24(12):191–200, 2022 36459387

Mekonnen AB, Abebe TB, McLachlan AJ, et al: Impact of electronic medication reconciliation interventions on medication discrepancies at hospital transitions: a systematic review and meta-analysis. BMC Med Inform Decis Mak 16(1):112, 2016a 27549581

Mekonnen AB, McLachlan AJ, Brien JA: Pharmacy-led medication reconciliation programmes at hospital transitions: a systematic review and meta-analysis. J Clin Pharm Ther 41(2):128–144, 2016b 26913812

Mevorach L, Forookhi A, Farcomeni A, et al: Perioperative risk factors associated with increased incidence of postoperative delirium: systematic review, meta-analysis, and Grading of Recommendations Assessment, Development, and Evaluation system report of clinical literature. Br J Anaesth 130(2):e254–e262, 2023 35810005

Meyer G, Mauch M, Seeger Y, et al: Experiences of relatives of patients with delirium due to an acute health event - a systematic review of qualitative studies. Appl Nurs Res 73:151722, 2023 37722790

Meyer-Massetti C, Cheng CM, Sharpe BA, et al: The FDA extended warning for intravenous haloperidol and torsades de pointes: how should institutions respond? J Hosp Med 5(4):E8–E16, 2010 20394022

Miarons M, Rofes L: Systematic review of case reports of oropharyngeal dysphagia following the use of antipsychotics. Gastroenterol Hepatol 42(4):209–227, 2019 30470564

Micromedex: Micromedex® (electronic version). Ann Arbor, MI, Merative, 2024. Available at: https://www.micromedexsolutions.com. Accessed August 16, 2024.

Mikkelsen ME, Still M, Anderson BJ, et al: Society of Critical Care Medicine's international consensus conference on prediction and identification of long-term impairments after critical illness. Crit Care Med 48(11):1670–1679, 2020 32947467

Minich DM, Henning M, Darley C, et al: Is melatonin the "Next Vitamin D"? A review of emerging science, clinical uses, safety, and dietary supplements. Nutrients 14(19):3934, 2022 36235587

Mion LC, Tan A, Brockman A, et al: An exploration of critical care professionals' strategies to enhance daily implementation of the Assess, prevent, and manage pain; Both spontaneous awakening and breathing trials; Choice of analgesia and sedation; Delirium assess, prevent, and manage; Early mobility and exercise; and Family engagement and empowerment: A group concept mapping study. Crit Care Explor 5(3):e0872, 2023 36890874

Mitchell AJ, Bird V, Rizzo M, et al: Diagnostic validity and added value of the Geriatric Depression Scale for depression in primary care: a meta-analysis of GDS30 and GDS15. J Affect Disord 125(1-3):10–17, 2010 19800132

Mohanty S, Rosenthal RA, Russell MM, et al: Optimal perioperative management of the geriatric patient: a best practices guideline from the American College of Surgeons NSQIP and the American Geriatrics Society. J Am Coll Surg 222(5):930–947, 2016 27049783

Moon E, Kim K, Partonen T, et al: Role of melatonin in the management of sleep and circadian disorders in the context of psychiatric illness. Curr Psychiatry Rep 24(11):623–634, 2022a 36227449

Moon E, Partonen T, Beaulieu S, Linnaranta O: Melatonergic agents influence the sleep-wake and circadian rhythms in healthy and psychiatric participants: a systematic review and meta-analysis of randomized controlled trials. Neuropsychopharmacology 47(8):1523–1536, 2022b 35115662

Moore C, Damari N, Liles EA, et al: Who you gonna call? Outcomes of a team-based approach to respond to disruptive behavioral issues in hospitalized patients. Jt Comm J Qual Patient Saf 45(11):781–785, 2019 31582223

Morandi A, McCurley J, Vasilevskis EE, et al: Tools to detect delirium superimposed on dementia: a systematic review [published erratum appears in J Am Geriatr Soc 61(1):174, 2013]. J Am Geriatr Soc 60(11):2005–2013, 2012 23039270

Morandi A, Davis D, Fick DM, et al: Delirium superimposed on dementia strongly predicts worse outcomes in older rehabilitation inpatients. J Am Med Dir Assoc 15(5):349–354, 2014 24566447

Moss MJ, Hendrickson RG; Toxicology Investigators Consortium (ToxIC): Serotonin toxicity: associated agents and clinical characteristics [published erratum appears in J Clin Psychopharmacol 41(2):226, 2021]. J Clin Psychopharmacol 39(6):628–633, 2019 31688388

Motyl CM, Ngo L, Zhou W, et al: Comparative accuracy and efficiency of four delirium screening protocols. J Am Geriatr Soc 68(11):2572–2578, 2020 32930409

Müller M, Jürgens J, Redaèlli M, et al: Impact of the communication and patient hand-off tool SBAR on patient safety: a systematic review. BMJ Open 8(8):e022202, 2018 30139905

Nagari N, Babu MS: Assessment of risk factors and precipitating factors of delirium in patients admitted to intensive care unit of a tertiary care hospital. British Journal of Medical Practitioners 12(2):a011, 2019

Nasreddine ZS, Phillips NA, Bédirian V, et al: The Montreal Cognitive Assessment, MoCA: a brief screening tool for mild cognitive impairment. J Am Geriatr Soc 53(4):695–699, 2005 15817019

National Institute for Health and Care Excellence: Delirium: Prevention, Diagnosis and Management in Hospital and Long-Term Care. London, National Institute for Health and Care Excellence, 2023. Available at: https://www.nice.org.uk/guidance/cg103/resources/delirium-prevention-diagnosis-and-management-in-hospital-and-longterm-care-pdf-35109327290821. Accessed December 5, 2023.

National Task Group on Intellectual Disabilities and Dementia Practices and the Health Matters Program: Over-Medication and Older Adults With Intellectual Disability: Risks for Brain Health. Rockport, Maine, National Task Group on Intellectual Disabilities and Dementia Practices, February 2023. Available at: https://www.the-ntg.org/_files/ugd/8c1d0a_4f34eb50cccb4e398b521764716c756c.pdf. Accessed July 21, 2024.

Nicolle LE: Urinary tract infections in the older adult. Clin Geriatr Med 32(3):523–538, 2016 27394021

Nicolle LE, Gupta K, Bradley SF, et al: Clinical practice guideline for the management of asymptomatic bacteriuria: 2019 update by the Infectious Diseases Society of America. Clin Infect Dis 68(10):e83–e110, 2019 30895288

Oberhaus J, Wang W, Mickle AM, et al: Evaluation of the 3-Minute Diagnostic Confusion Assessment Method for identification of postoperative delirium in older patients. JAMA Netw Open 4(12):e2137267, 2021 34902038

Oh ES, Fong TG, Hshieh TT, et al: Delirium in older persons: advances in diagnosis and treatment. JAMA 318(12):1161–1174, 2017 28973626

Oh ST, Park JY: Postoperative delirium. Korean J Anesthesiol 72(1):4–12, 2019 30139213

Oldham MA, Lee HB: Catatonia vis-à-vis delirium: the significance of recognizing catatonia in altered mental status. Gen Hosp Psychiatry 37(6):554–559, 2015 26162545

Oldham MA, Flaherty JH, Rudolph JL: Debating the role of arousal in delirium diagnosis: should delirium diagnosis be inclusive or restrictive? J Am Med Dir Assoc 18(7):629–631, 2017 28442228

Oliveira J E Silva L, Berning MJ, Stanich JA, et al: Risk factors for delirium in older adults in the emergency department: a systematic review and meta-analysis. Ann Emerg Med 78(4):549–565, 2021 34127307

O'Mahony D, O'Sullivan D, Byrne S, et al: STOPP/START criteria for potentially inappropriate prescribing in older people: version 2. Age Ageing 44(2):213–218, 2015 25324330

O'Regan NA, Fitzgerald J, Adamis D, et al: Predictors of delirium development in older medical inpatients: readily identifiable factors at admission. J Alzheimers Dis 64(3):775–785, 2018 29966197

Ormseth CH, LaHue SC, Oldham MA, et al: Predisposing and precipitating factors associated with delirium: a systematic review. JAMA Netw Open 6(1):e2249950, 2023 36607634

O'Rourke G, Parker D, Anderson R, et al: Interventions to support recovery following an episode of delirium: a realist synthesis. Aging Ment Health 25(10):1769–1785, 2021 32734773

Ospina JP, King F IV, Madva E, et al: Epidemiology, mechanisms, diagnosis, and treatment of delirium: a narrative review. Clin Med Ther 1(1):3, 2018

Ouimet S, Kavanagh BP, Gottfried SB, et al: Incidence, risk factors and consequences of ICU delirium. Intensive Care Med 33(1):66–73, 2007 17102966

Palihnich K, Gallagher J, Inouye SK, et al: The 3D CAM Training Manual for Research, Version 5.5. Boston, MA, Beth Israel Deaconess Medical Center, 2023

Pandhal JK, Van Der Wardt V: Exploring perceptions regarding family-based delirium management in the intensive care unit. J Intensive Care Soc 23(4):447–452, 2022 36751350

Pandharipande PP, Girard TD, Jackson JC, et al; BRAIN-ICU Study Investigators: Long-term cognitive impairment after critical illness. N Engl J Med 369(14):1306–1316, 2013 24088092

Pathan S, Kaplan JB, Adamczyk K, et al: Evaluation of dexmedetomidine withdrawal in critically ill adults. J Crit Care 62:19–24, 2021 33227592

Peel NM, Hornby-Turner YC, Henderson A, et al: Prevalence and impact of functional and psychosocial problems in hospitalized adults: a prospective cohort study. J Am Med Dir Assoc 20(10):1294–1299.e1, 2019 31078487

Penfold RS, Squires C, Angus A, et al: Delirium detection tools show varying completion rates and positive score rates when used at scale in routine practice in general hospital settings: a systematic review. J Am Geriatr Soc 72(5):1508–1524, 2024 38241503

Pereira JV, Aung Thein MZ, Nitchingham A, et al: Delirium in older adults is associated with development of new dementia: a systematic review and meta-analysis. Int J Geriatr Psychiatry 36(7):993–1003, 2021 33638566

Perez D, Peters K, Wilkes L, et al: Physical restraints in intensive care: an integrative review. Aust Crit Care 32(2):165–174, 2019 29559190

Perez D, Murphy G, Wilkes L, et al: Being tied down: the experience of being physically restrained while mechanically ventilated in ICU. J Adv Nurs 78(11):3760–3771, 2022 35789502

Peterson A, Marengoni A, Shenkin S, et al: Delirium in COVID-19: common, distressing and linked with poor outcomes. . . can we do better? Age Ageing 50(5):1436–1438, 2021 34174069

Pisani MA, Redlich C, McNicoll L, et al: Underrecognition of preexisting cognitive impairment by physicians in older ICU patients. Chest 124(6):2267–2274, 2003 14665510

Pisani MA, Murphy TE, Van Ness PH, et al: Characteristics associated with delirium in older patients in a medical intensive care unit. Arch Intern Med 167(15):1629–1634, 2007 17698685

Potter J, George J; Guideline Development Group: The prevention, diagnosis and management of delirium in older people: concise guidelines. Clin Med (Lond) 6(3):303–308, 2006 16826866

Pottie K, Thompson W, Davies S, et al: Deprescribing benzodiazepine receptor agonists: evidence-based clinical practice guideline. Can Fam Physician 64(5):339–351, 2018 29760253

Prendergast NT, Tiberio PJ, Girard TD: Treatment of delirium during critical illness. Annu Rev Med 73:407–421, 2022 34752706

Preskorn SH, Zeller S, Citrome L, et al: Effect of sublingual dexmedetomidine vs placebo on acute agitation associated with bipolar disorder: a randomized clinical trial. JAMA 327(8):727–736, 2022 35191924

Procyshyn RM, Bezchlibnyk-Butler KZ, Kim DD (eds): Clinical Handbook of Psychotropic Drugs, 25th Edition. Newburyport, MA, Hogrefe, 2023. Available at: https://chpd.hogrefe.com. Accessed December 4, 2023.

Pugh RN, Murray-Lyon IM, Dawson JL, et al: Transection of the oesophagus for bleeding oesophageal varices. Br J Surg 60(8):646–649, 1973 4541913

Pun BT, Balas MC, Barnes-Daly MA, et al: Caring for critically ill patients with the ABCDEF bundle: results of the ICU Liberation Collaborative in over 15,000 adults. Crit Care Med 47(1):3–14, 2019 30339549

Pun BT, Badenes R, Heras La Calle G, et al; COVID-19 Intensive Care International Study Group: Prevalence and risk factors for delirium in critically ill patients with COVID-19 (COVID-D): a multicentre cohort study. Lancet Respir Med 9(3):239–250, 2021 33428871

Quispel-Aggenbach DWP, Schep-de Ruiter EPR, van Bergen W, et al: Prevalence and risk factors of delirium in psychogeriatric outpatients. Int J Geriatr Psychiatry 36(1):190–196, 2021 32844507

Rahman S, Byatt K: Follow-up services for delirium after COVID-19—where now? Age Ageing 50(3):601–604, 2021 33951153

Ramnarain D, Pouwels S, Fernández-Gonzalo S, et al: Delirium-related psychiatric and neurocognitive impairment and the association with post-intensive care syndrome: a narrative review. Acta Psychiatr Scand 147(5):460–474, 2023 36744298

Redmond P, Grimes TC, McDonnell R, et al: Impact of medication reconciliation for improving transitions of care. Cochrane Database Syst Rev 8(8):CD010791, 2018 30136718

Reeve E: Deprescribing tools: a review of the types of tools available to aid deprescribing in clinical practice. J Pharm Pract Res 50:98–107, 2020

Registered Nurses' Association of Ontario: Delirium, Dementia, and Depression in Older Adults: Assessment and Care, 2nd Edition. Toronto, ON, Canada, Registered Nurses' Association of Ontario, 2016. Available at: https://rnao.ca/bpg/guidelines/assessment-and-care-older-adults-delirium-dementia-and-depression. Accessed December 5, 2023.

Reisinger M, Reininghaus EZ, Biasi J, et al: Delirium-associated medication in people at risk: a systematic update review, meta-analyses, and GRADE-profiles. Acta Psychiatr Scand 147(1):16–42, 2023 36168988

Rengel KF, Hayhurst CJ, Jackson JC, et al: Motoric subtypes of delirium and long-term functional and mental health outcomes in adults after critical illness. Crit Care Med 49(5):e521–e532, 2021 33729717

Reppas-Rindlisbacher C, Shin S, Purohit U, et al: Association between non-English language and use of physical and chemical restraints among medical inpatients with delirium. J Am Geriatr Soc 70(12):3640–3643, 2022 35932190

Richardson SJ, Davis DHJ, Stephan BCM, et al: Recurrent delirium over 12 months predicts dementia: results of the Delirium and Cognitive Impact in Dementia (DECIDE) study. Age Ageing 50(3):914–920, 2021 33320945

Richmond JS, Berlin JS, Fishkind AB, et al: Verbal de-escalation of the agitated patient: consensus statement of the American Association for Emergency Psychiatry Project BETA De-escalation Workgroup. West J Emerg Med 13(1):17–25, 2012 22461917

Rinehart MC, Ghorashi S, Heavner MS, et al: An assessment of a sleep aid and sleep promotion practices in hospitalized medical patients. J Am Pharm Assoc (2003) 64(3):102042, 2024 38382836

Risperdal (risperidone) [product monograph]. Toronto, ON, Canada, Janssen, Inc, December 2020

Risperdal (risperidone) [prescribing information]. Titusville, NJ, Janssen Pharmaceuticals, Inc, March 2022

Risperidone orally disintegrating tablets (risperidone) [prescribing information]. Princeton, NJ, Sandoz, Inc, February 2019

Robinson L, Cramer LD, Ray JM, et al: Racial and ethnic disparities in use of chemical restraint in the emergency department. Acad Emerg Med 29(12):1496–1499, 2022 35934988

Roerig JL, Steffen K: Psychopharmacology and bariatric surgery. Eur Eat Disord Rev 23(6):463–469, 2015 26338011

Rogers JP, Oldham MA, Fricchione G, et al: Evidence-based consensus guidelines for the management of catatonia: recommendations from the British Association for Psychopharmacology. J Psychopharmacol 37(4):327–369, 2023 37039129

Rood PJT, van de Schoor F, van Tertholen K, et al: Differences in 90-day mortality of delirium subtypes in the intensive care unit: a retrospective cohort study. J Crit Care 53:120–124, 2019 31228762

Roppolo LP, Morris DW, Khan F, et al: Improving the management of acutely agitated patients in the emergency department through implementation of Project BETA (Best Practices in the Evaluation and Treatment of Agitation). J Am Coll Emerg Physicians Open 1(5):898–907, 2020 33145538

Rose L, Burry L, Mallick R, et al: Prevalence, risk factors, and outcomes associated with physical restraint use in mechanically ventilated adults. J Crit Care 31(1):31–35, 2016 26489482

Rosenthal JL, Doiron R, Haynes SC, et al: The effectiveness of standardized handoff tool interventions during inter- and intra-facility care transitions on patient-related outcomes: a systematic review. Am J Med Qual 33(2):193–206, 2018 28467104

Rosgen BK, Krewulak KD, Davidson JE, et al: Associations between caregiver-detected delirium and symptoms of depression and anxiety in family caregivers of critically ill patients: a cross-sectional study. BMC Psychiatry 21(1):187, 2021 33836699

Rungvivatjarus T, Kuelbs CL, Miller L, et al: Medication reconciliation improvement utilizing process redesign and clinical decision support. Jt Comm J Qual Patient Saf 46(1):27–36, 2020 31653526

Rush AJ, First MB, Blacker D (eds): Handbook of Psychiatric Measures, 2nd Edition. Washington, DC, American Psychiatric Publishing, 2008

Ryan DJ, O'Regan NA, Caoimh RÓ, et al: Delirium in an adult acute hospital population: predictors, prevalence and detection. BMJ Open 3(1):e001772, 2013 23299110

Ryan SL, Kimchi EY: Evaluation and management of delirium. Semin Neurol 41(5):572–587, 2021 34619782

Saljuqi AT, Hanna K, Asmar S, et al: Prospective evaluation of delirium in geriatric patients undergoing emergency general surgery. J Am Coll Surg 230(5):758–765, 2020 32088308

Salluh JI, Wang H, Schneider EB, et al: Outcome of delirium in critically ill patients: systematic review and meta-analysis. BMJ 350:h2538, 2015 26041151

Sanchez D, Brennan K, Al Sayfe M, et al: Frailty, delirium and hospital mortality of older adults admitted to intensive care: the Delirium (Deli) in ICU study. Crit Care 24(1):609, 2020 33059749

Sandson NB, Armstrong SC, Cozza KL: An overview of psychotropic drug-drug interactions. Psychosomatics 46(5):464–494, 2005 16145193

Sateia MJ, Buysse DJ, Krystal AD, et al: Clinical practice guideline for the pharmacologic treatment of chronic insomnia in adults: an American Academy of Sleep Medicine Clinical Practice Guideline. J Clin Sleep Med 13(2):307–349, 2017 27998379

Sawan M, Reeve E, Turner J, et al: A systems approach to identifying the challenges of implementing deprescribing in older adults across different health-care settings and countries: a narrative review. Expert Rev Clin Pharmacol 13(3):233–245, 2020 32056451

Schneider-Thoma J, Efthimiou O, Huhn M, et al: Second-generation antipsychotic drugs and short-term mortality: a systematic review and meta-analysis of placebo-controlled randomised controlled trials. Lancet Psychiatry 5(8):653–663, 2018 30042077

Schnipper JL, Reyes Nieva H, Mallouk M, et al; MARQUIS2 Site Leaders; MARQUIS2 Study Group: Effects of a refined evidence-based toolkit and mentored implementation on medication reconciliation at 18 hospitals: results of the MARQUIS2 study. BMJ Qual Saf 31(4):278–286, 2022 33927025

Schnipper JL, Reyes Nieva H, Yoon C, et al; MARQUIS2 Site Leaders for the MARQUIS2 Study Group; MARQUIS2 Site Leaders: What works in medication reconciliation: an on-treatment and site analysis of the MARQUIS2 study. BMJ Qual Saf 32(8):457–469, 2023 36948542

Schnitzer K, Merideth F, Macias-Konstantopoulos W, et al: Disparities in care: the role of race on the utilization of physical restraints in the emergency setting. Acad Emerg Med 27(10):943–950, 2020 32691509

Schofield-Robinson OJ, Lewis SR, Smith AF, et al: Follow-up services for improving long-term outcomes in intensive care unit (ICU) survivors. Cochrane Database Syst Rev 11(11):CD012701, 2018 30388297

Scott IA, Reeve E, Hilmer SN: Establishing the worth of deprescribing inappropriate medications: are we there yet? Med J Aust 217(6):283–286, 2022 36030510

Scottish Intercollegiate Guidelines Network (SIGN): Risk Reduction and Management of Delirium: A National Clinical Guideline (SIGN Publ No 157). Edinburgh, UK, Scottish Intercollegiate Guidelines Network, 2019. Available at: https://www.sign.ac.uk/media/1423/sign157.pdf. Accessed December 5, 2023.

Semple D, Howlett MM, Strawbridge JD, et al: A systematic review and pooled prevalence of delirium in critically ill children. Crit Care Med 50(2):317–328, 2022 34387241

Sepulveda E, Franco JG, Trzepacz PT, et al: Performance of the Delirium Rating Scale-Revised-98 against different delirium diagnostic criteria in a population with a high prevalence of dementia. Psychosomatics 56(5):530–541, 2015 26278338

Sepulveda E, Leonard M, Franco JG, et al: Subsyndromal delirium compared with delirium, dementia, and subjects without delirium or dementia in elderly general hospital admissions and nursing home residents. Alzheimers Dement (Amst) 7:1–10, 2016 28116342

Sepúlveda E, Bermúdez E, González D, et al: Validation of the Delirium Diagnostic Tool-Provisional (DDT-Pro) in a skilled nursing facility and comparison to the 4 'A's test (4AT). Gen Hosp Psychiatry 70:116–123, 2021 33813146

Seroquel (quetiapine) [prescribing information]. Wilmington, DE, AstraZeneca Pharmaceuticals LP, January 2022

Seroquel XR (quetiapine extended release) [prescribing information]. Wilmington, DE, AstraZeneca Pharmaceuticals LP, January 2022

Sharifi A, Arsalani N, Fallahi-Khoshknab M, et al: The principles of physical restraint use for hospitalized elderly people: an integrated literature review. Syst Rev 10(1):129, 2021 33931096

Shehabi Y, Serpa Neto A, Howe BD, et al; SPICE III Study Investigators: Early sedation with dexmedetomidine in ventilated critically ill patients and heterogeneity of treatment effect in the SPICE III randomised controlled trial. Intensive Care Med 47(4):455–466, 2021 33686482

Sheikh JI, Yesavage JA: Geriatric Depression Scale (GDS): recent evidence and development of a shorter version, in Clinical Gerontology: A Guide to Assessment and Intervention. Edited by Brink TL. New York, Haworth, 1986, pp 165–173

Shenkin SD, Fox C, Godfrey M, et al: Delirium detection in older acute medical inpatients: a multicentre prospective comparative diagnostic test accuracy study of the 4AT and the confusion assessment method. BMC Med 17(1):138, 2019 31337404

Shenvi C, Kennedy M, Austin CA, et al: Managing delirium and agitation in the older emergency department patient: The ADEPT tool. Ann Emerg Med 75(2):136–145, 2020 31563402

Showler L, Ali Abdelhamid Y, Goldin J, et al: Sleep during and following critical illness: a narrative review. World J Crit Care Med 12(3):92–115, 2023 37397589

Shrestha P, Fick DM: Family caregiver's experience of caring for an older adult with delirium: a systematic review. Int J Older People Nurs 15(4):e12321, 2020 32374518

Silver GH, Kearney JA, Bora S, et al; PATHWAYS FOR CLINICAL CARE WORKGROUP: A clinical pathway to standardize care of children with delirium in pediatric inpatient settings. Hosp Pediatr 9(11):909–916, 2019 31662421

Simpson N: Delirium in adults with intellectual disabilities and DC-LD. J Intellect Disabil Res 47(Suppl 1):38–42, 2003 14516372

Singh A, Gupta I, Wright SM, et al: Outcomes among hospitalized patients with dementia and behavioral disturbances when physical restraints are introduced. J Am Geriatr Soc 71(9):2886–2892, 2023 37235512

Slooter AJC, Otte WM, Devlin JW, et al: Updated nomenclature of delirium and acute encephalopathy: statement of ten societies. Intensive Care Med 46(5):1020–1022, 2020 32055887

Smith CM, Turner NA, Thielman NM, et al: Association of Black race with physical and chemical restraint use among patients undergoing emergency psychiatric evaluation. Psychiatr Serv 73(7):730–736, 2022 34932385

Smith HAB, Besunder JB, Betters KA, et al: 2022 Society of Critical Care Medicine clinical practice guidelines on prevention and management of pain, agitation, neuromuscular blockade, and delirium in critically ill pediatric patients with consideration of the ICU environment and early mobility. Pediatr Crit Care Med 23(2):e74–e110, 2022 35119438

Smithard D, Randhawa R: Physical restraint in the critical care unit: a narrative review. New Bioeth 28(1):68–82, 2022 35083967

Society of Critical Care Medicine: ICU Liberation. Mount Prospect, IL, Society of Critical Care Medicine, 2023. Available at: https://www.sccm.org//ICULiberation/Home. Accessed September 27, 2023.

Sosnowski K, Lin F, Chaboyer W, et al: The effect of the ABCDE/ABCDEF bundle on delirium, functional outcomes, and quality of life in critically ill patients: a systematic review and meta-analysis. Int J Nurs Stud 138:104410, 2023 36577261

Spiropoulou E, Samanidis G, Kanakis M, et al: Risk factors for acute postoperative delirium in cardiac surgery patients >65 years old. J Pers Med 12(9):1529, 2022 36143313

Spitzer RL, Kroenke K, Williams JB, et al: A brief measure for assessing generalized anxiety disorder: the GAD-7. Arch Intern Med 166(10):1092–1097, 2006 16717171

Spronk PE, Riekerk B, Hofhuis J, et al: Occurrence of delirium is severely underestimated in the ICU during daily care. Intensive Care Med 35(7):1276–1280, 2009 19350214

SteelFisher GK, Martin LA, Dowal SL, et al: Sustaining clinical programs during difficult economic times: a case series from the Hospital Elder Life Program. J Am Geriatr Soc 59(10):1873–1882, 2011 22091501

SteelFisher GK, Martin LA, Dowal SL, et al: Learning from the closure of clinical programs: a case series from the Hospital Elder Life Program. J Am Geriatr Soc 61(6):999–1004, 2013 23730748

Stollings JL, Boncyk CS, Birdrow CI, et al: Antipsychotics and the QTc interval during delirium in the intensive care unit: a secondary analysis of a randomized clinical trial. JAMA Netw Open 7(1):e2352034, 2024 38252439

Strawn JR, Keck PE Jr, Caroff SN: Neuroleptic malignant syndrome. Am J Psychiatry 164(6):870–876, 2007 17541044

Stroomer-van Wijk AJ, Jonker BW, Kok RM, et al: Detecting delirium in elderly outpatients with cognitive impairment. Int Psychogeriatr 28(8):1303–1311, 2016 27079735

Stuart MM, Smith ZR, Payter KA, et al: Pharmacist-driven discontinuation of antipsychotics for ICU delirium: a quasi-experimental study. J Am Coll Clin Pharm 3(6):1009–1014, 2020

Tamblyn R, Abrahamowicz M, Buckeridge DL, et al: Effect of an electronic medication reconciliation intervention on adverse drug events: a cluster randomized trial. JAMA Netw Open 2(9):e1910756, 2019 31539073

Tanwani R, Danquah MO, Butris N, et al: Diagnostic accuracy of Ascertain Dementia 8-item Questionnaire by participant and informant: a systematic review and meta-analysis. PLoS One 18(9):e0291291, 2023 37699028

Tariq SH, Tumosa N, Chibnall JT, et al: Comparison of the Saint Louis University mental status examination and the mini-mental state examination for detecting dementia and mild neurocognitive disorder—a pilot study. Am J Geriatr Psychiatry 14(11):900–910, 2006 17068312

Teece A, Baker J, Smith H: Identifying determinants for the application of physical or chemical restraint in the management of psychomotor agitation on the critical care unit. J Clin Nurs 29(1-2):5–19, 2020 31495002

Theisen-Toupal J, Breu AC, Mattison ML, et al: Diagnostic yield of head computed tomography for the hospitalized medical patient with delirium. J Hosp Med 9(8):497–501, 2014 24733711

The Joint Commission: Diagnostic overshadowing among groups experiencing health disparities. Sentinel Event Alert (65):1–7, 2022

The WHOQOL Group: Development of the World Health Organization WHOQOL-BREF quality of life assessment. Psychol Med 28(3):551–558, 1998a 9626712

The WHOQOL Group: The World Health Organization Quality of Life Assessment (WHOQOL): development and general psychometric properties. Soc Sci Med 46(12):1569–1585, 1998b 9672396

Thom RP, Levy-Carrick NC, Bui M, et al: Delirium. Am J Psychiatry 176(10):785–793, 2019 31569986

Tieges Z, Maclullich AMJ, Anand A, et al: Diagnostic accuracy of the 4AT for delirium detection in older adults: systematic review and meta-analysis. Age Ageing 50(3):733–743, 2021 33951145

Tornio A, Filppula AM, Niemi M, et al: Clinical studies on drug-drug interactions involving metabolism and transport: methodology, pitfalls, and interpretation. Clin Pharmacol Ther 105(6):1345–1361, 2019 30916389

Trifirò G, Spina E: Age-related changes in pharmacodynamics: focus on drugs acting on central nervous and cardiovascular systems. Curr Drug Metab 12(7):611–620, 2011 21495972

Tropea J, Slee JA, Brand CA, et al: Clinical practice guidelines for the management of delirium in older people in Australia. Australas J Ageing 27(3):150–156, 2008 18713175

Trzepacz PT, Mittal D, Torres R, et al: Validation of the Delirium Rating Scale-Revised-98: comparison with the delirium rating scale and the cognitive test for delirium. J Neuropsychiatry Clin Neurosci 13(2):229–242, 2001 11449030

Trzepacz PT, Bourne R, Zhang S: Designing clinical trials for the treatment of delirium. J Psychosom Res 65(3):299–307, 2008 18707954

Trzepacz PT, Franco JG, Meagher DJ, et al: Phenotype of subsyndromal delirium using pooled multicultural Delirium Rating Scale—Revised-98 data. J Psychosom Res 73(1):10–17, 2012 22691554

Tsai YV, Fawzy JH, Durkin JB, et al: Off-label use of intravenous olanzapine for agitation after neurologic injury. Hosp Pharm 56(6):697–701, 2021 34732924

Tse AHW, Ling L, Lee A, et al: Altered pharmacokinetics in prolonged infusions of sedatives and analgesics among adult critically ill patients: a systematic review. Clin Ther 40(9):1598–1615.e2, 2018 30173953

Tsui A, Searle SD, Bowden H, et al: The effect of baseline cognition and delirium on long-term cognitive impairment and mortality: a prospective population-based study. Lancet Healthy Longev 3(4):e232–e241, 2022 35382093

U.S. Food and Drug Administration: Public Health Advisory: Deaths With Antipsychotics in Elderly Patients With Behavioral Disturbances. Silver Spring, MD, U.S. Food and Drug Administration, 2005. Available at: https://wayback.archive-it.org/7993/20170113112252/http://www.fda.gov/Drugs/DrugSafety/PostmarketDrugSafetyInformationforPatientsandProviders/ucm053171.htm. Accessed October 22, 2023.

U.S. Food and Drug Administration: Information for Healthcare Professionals: Conventional Antipsychotics. Silver Spring, MD, U.S. Food and Drug Administration, 2008. Available at: https://wayback.archive-it.org/7993/20170722190727/https://www.fda.gov/Drugs/DrugSafety/PostmarketDrugSafetyInformationforPatientsandProviders/ucm124830.htm. Accessed October 22, 2023.

U.S. Preventive Services Task Force; Mangione CM, Barry MJ, Nicholson WK, et al: Screening for syphilis infection in nonpregnant adolescents and adults: US Preventive Services Task Force Reaffirmation Recommendation Statement. JAMA 328(12):1243–1249, 2022 36166020

Vacas S, Grogan T, Cheng D, et al: Risk factor stratification for postoperative delirium: a retrospective database study. Medicine (Baltimore) 101(42):e31176, 2022 36281117

Valtis YK, Stevenson KE, Murphy EM, et al: Race and ethnicity and the utilization of security responses in a hospital setting. J Gen Intern Med 38(1):30–35, 2023 35556213

van den Boogaard M, Schoonhoven L, Evers AW, et al: Delirium in critically ill patients: impact on long-term health-related quality of life and cognitive functioning. Crit Care Med 40(1):112–118, 2012 21926597

van den Boogaard M, Wassenaar A, van Haren FMP, et al: Influence of sedation on delirium recognition in critically ill patients: a multinational cohort study. Aust Crit Care 33(5):420–425, 2020 32035691

van den Boogaard M, Leenders M, Pop-Purceleanu M, et al: Performance and validation of two ICU delirium assessment and severity tools; a prospective observational study. Intensive Crit Care Nurs 83:103627, 2024 38301387

van Eijk MM, van den Boogaard M, van Marum RJ, et al: Routine use of the confusion assessment method for the intensive care unit: a multicenter study. Am J Respir Crit Care Med 184(3):340–344, 2011 21562131

van Rensburg R, Decloedt EH: An approach to the pharmacotherapy of neuroleptic malignant syndrome. Psychopharmacol Bull 49(1):84–91, 2019 30858642

van Velthuijsen EL, Zwakhalen SM, Warnier RM, et al: Psychometric properties and feasibility of instruments for the detection of delirium in older hospitalized patients: a systematic review. Int J Geriatr Psychiatry 31(9):974–989, 2016 26898375

van Velthuijsen EL, Zwakhalen SMG, Pijpers E, et al: Effects of a medication review on delirium in older hospitalised patients: a comparative retrospective cohort study. Drugs Aging 35(2):153–161, 2018 29396715
Van Waarde JA, Van Der Mast RC: Delirium in learning disability: case series and literature review. Br J Learn Disabil 32:123–127, 2004
Vasilevskis EE, Han JH, Hughes CG, et al: Epidemiology and risk factors for delirium across hospital settings. Best Pract Res Clin Anaesthesiol 26(3):277–287, 2012 23040281
Vasilevskis EE, Chandrasekhar R, Holtze CH, et al: The cost of ICU delirium and coma in the intensive care unit patient. Med Care 56(10):890–897, 2018 30179988
Vasunilashorn SM, Guess J, Ngo L, et al: Derivation and validation of a severity scoring method for the 3-Minute Diagnostic Interview for Confusion Assessment Method--Defined Delirium. J Am Geriatr Soc 64(8):1684–1689, 2016 27374833
Visser L, Prent A, Banning LBD, et al: Risk factors for delirium after vascular surgery: a systematic review and meta-analysis. Ann Vasc Surg 76:500–513, 2021 33905851
Walia H, Tucker LS, Manickam RN, et al: Patient and visit characteristics associated with physical restraint use in the emergency department. Perm J 27(1):94–102, 2023 36464780
Wang E, Belley-Côté EP, Young J, et al: Effect of perioperative benzodiazepine use on intraoperative awareness and postoperative delirium: a systematic review and meta-analysis of randomised controlled trials and observational studies. Br J Anaesth 131(2):302–313, 2023 36621439
Wang M, Yankama TT, Abdallah GT, et al: A retrospective comparison of the effectiveness and safety of intravenous olanzapine versus intravenous haloperidol for agitation in adult intensive care unit patients. J Intensive Care Med 37(2):222–230, 2022 33426981
Weerink MAS, Struys MMRF, Hannivoort LN, et al: Clinical pharmacokinetics and pharmacodynamics of dexmedetomidine. Clin Pharmacokinet 56(8):893–913, 2017 28105598
Wei LA, Fearing MA, Sternberg EJ, et al: The Confusion Assessment Method: a systematic review of current usage. J Am Geriatr Soc 56(5):823–830, 2008 18384586
Weidman K, LaFond E, Hoffman KL, et al: Post-intensive care unit syndrome in a cohort of COVID-19 survivors in New York City. Ann Am Thorac Soc 19(7):1158–1168, 2022 34936536
Weinrebe W, Johannsdottir E, Karaman M, et al: What does delirium cost? An economic evaluation of hyperactive delirium. Z Gerontol Geriatr 49(1):52–58, 2016 25801513
Welk B, Killin L, Reid JN, et al: Effect of electronic medication reconciliation at the time of hospital discharge on inappropriate medication use in the community: an interrupted time-series analysis. CMAJ Open 9(4):E1105–E1113, 2021 34848551
White B, Snyder HS, Patel MVB: Evaluation of medications used for hospitalized patients with sleep disturbances: a frequency analysis and literature review. J Pharm Pract 36(1):126–138, 2023 34096384
Wilcox ME, Girard TD, Hough CL: Delirium and long term cognition in critically ill patients. BMJ 373:n1007, 2021 34103334
Wilke V, Sulyok M, Stefanou MI, et al: Delirium in hospitalized COVID-19 patients: predictors and implications for patient outcome. PLoS One 17(12):e0278214, 2022 36548347
Williams ST, Dhesi JK, Partridge JSL: Distress in delirium: causes, assessment and management. Eur Geriatr Med 11(1):63–70, 2020 32297237
Wilson JE, Carlson R, Duggan MC, et al; Delirium and Catatonia (DeCat) Prospective Cohort Investigation: Delirium and catatonia in critically ill patients: the delirium and catatonia prospective cohort investigation. Crit Care Med 45(11):1837–1844, 2017 28841632
Wilson JE, Mart MF, Cunningham C, et al: Delirium. Nat Rev Dis Primers 6(1):90, 2020 33184265
Wilson MP, Pepper D, Currier GW, et al: The psychopharmacology of agitation: consensus statement of the American Association for Emergency Psychiatry Project Beta Psychopharmacology Workgroup. West J Emerg Med 13(1):26–34, 2012 22461918
Wolters AE, van Dijk D, Pasma W, et al: Long-term outcome of delirium during intensive care unit stay in survivors of critical illness: a prospective cohort study. Crit Care 18(3):R125, 2014 24942154
Wolters AE, Peelen LM, Welling MC, et al: Long-term mental health problems after delirium in the ICU. Crit Care Med 44(10):1808–1813, 2016 27513540
Wong AH, Ray JM, Rosenberg A, et al: Experiences of individuals who were physically restrained in the emergency department. JAMA Netw Open 3(1):e1919381, 2020 31977058
Wong AH, Whitfill T, Ohuabunwa EC, et al: Association of race/ethnicity and other demographic characteristics with use of physical restraints in the emergency department. JAMA Netw Open 4(1):e2035241, 2021 33492372
Wong EK, Watt J, Zou H, et al: Characteristics, treatment and delirium incidence of older adults hospitalized with COVID-19: a multicentre retrospective cohort study. CMAJ Open 10(3):E692–E701, 2022 35882392
World Health Organization: Measuring Health and Disability: Manual for WHO Disability Assessment Schedule (WHODAS 2.0). Edited by Üstün TB, Kostanjesek N, Chatterji S, et al. Geneva, World Health Organization Press, 2010. Available at: https://www.who.int/publications/i/item/measuring-health-and-disability-manual-for-who-disability-assessment-schedule-(-whodas-2.0). Accessed July 23, 2022.
Wu CS, Wang SC, Yeh IJ, et al: Comparative risk of seizure with use of first- and second-generation antipsychotics in patients with schizophrenia and mood disorders. J Clin Psychiatry 77(5):e573–e579, 2016 27249081
Wu TT, Zegers M, Kooken R, et al: Social determinants of health and delirium occurrence and duration in critically ill adults. Crit Care Explor 3(9):e0532, 2021 34514427
Wu Y, Wang G, Zhang Z, et al: Efficacy and safety of unrestricted visiting policy for critically ill patients: a meta-analysis. Crit Care 26(1):267, 2022 36064613

Yap CYL, Taylor DM, Kong DCM, et al; Sedation for Acute Agitation in Emergency Department Patients: Targeting Adverse Events (SIESTA) Collaborative Study Group: Risk factors for sedation-related events during acute agitation management in the emergency department. Acad Emerg Med 26(10):1135–1143, 2019 31265756

Yesavage JA, Brink TL, Rose TL, et al: Development and validation of a geriatric depression screening scale: a preliminary report. J Psychiatr Res 17(1):37–49, 1982–1983 7183759

Yu D-N, Zhu Y, Ma J, et al: Comparison of post-anesthesia delirium in elderly patients treated with dexmedetomidine and midazolam maleate after thoracic surgery. Biomed Res 28(15):6852–6855, 2017

Yunusa I, Alsumali A, Garba AE, et al: Assessment of reported comparative effectiveness and safety of atypical antipsychotics in the treatment of behavioral and psychological symptoms of dementia: a network meta-analysis. JAMA Netw Open 2(3):e190828, 2019 30901041

Zaal IJ, Devlin JW, Peelen LM, et al: A systematic review of risk factors for delirium in the ICU. Crit Care Med 43(1):40–47, 2015 25251759

Zaman H, Gibson RC, Walcott G: Benzodiazepines for catatonia in people with schizophrenia or other serious mental illnesses. Cochrane Database Syst Rev 8(8):CD006570, 2019 31425609

Zeilinger EL, Zrnic Novakovic I, Komenda S, et al: Informant-based assessment instruments for dementia in people with intellectual disability: a systematic review and standardised evaluation. Res Dev Disabil 121:104148, 2022 34954669

Zghidi M, Saida IB, Kortli S, et al: Risk factors of post-traumatic stress disorder (PTSD) among ICU survivors. Ann Intensive Care 2019:1–153, 2019

Zhang H, Yuan J, Chen Q, et al: Development and validation of a predictive score for ICU delirium in critically ill patients. BMC Anesthesiol 21(1):37, 2021 33546592

Zhao S, Zhou R, Zhong Q, et al: Effect of age and ICU types on mortality in invasive mechanically ventilated patients with sepsis receiving dexmedetomidine: a retrospective cohort study with propensity score matching. Front Pharmacol 15:1344327, 2024 38487173

Zigmond AS, Snaith RP: The Hospital Anxiety and Depression Scale. Acta Psychiatr Scand 67(6):361–370, 1983 6880820

Zipser CM, Deuel J, Ernst J, et al: Predisposing and precipitating factors for delirium in neurology: a prospective cohort study of 1487 patients. J Neurol 266(12):3065–3075, 2019a 31520105

Zipser CM, Deuel J, Ernst J, et al: The predisposing and precipitating risk factors for delirium in neurosurgery: a prospective cohort study of 949 patients. Acta Neurochir (Wien) 161(7):1307–1315, 2019b 31106393

Zipser CM, Hildenbrand FF, Haubner B, et al: Predisposing and precipitating risk factors for delirium in elderly patients admitted to a cardiology ward: an observational cohort study in 1,042 patients. Front Cardiovasc Med 8:686665, 2021 34660708

Zyprexa (olanzapine) [prescribing information]. Indianapolis, IN, Lilly USA, LLC, February 2021

Disclosures

The Guideline Writing Group and Systematic Review Group reported the following disclosures during the development and approval of this guideline:

Catherine Crone, M.D., was employed by Inova Health Systems as Vice-Chair of Education, Department of Psychiatry, George Washington University/Inova Consultation-Liaison Psychiatry Fellowship Program Director, and Director of the Psychiatry Consult Service at Inova Fairfax Hospital. She is currently employed by Lyra Health and is Clinical Associate Professor at George Washington University Department of Psychiatry and Behavioral Sciences. She reports no conflicts of interest pertaining to her participation in the development of this guideline.

Laura J. Fochtmann, M.D., M.B.I., is employed as a Distinguished Service Professor of Psychiatry, Pharmacological Sciences, and Biomedical Informatics at Stony Brook University and as Deputy Chief Medical Information Officer for Stony Brook Medicine. She has been a co-investigator on a grant funded by the National Institute of Mental Health (NIMH). She also consults for the American Psychiatric Association (APA) on the development of practice guidelines and has received travel funds to attend meetings related to these duties.

Iqbal Ahmed, M.D., is a Clinical Professor of Psychiatry at the Uniformed Services University for Health Sciences and a Clinical Professor of Psychiatry and Geriatric Medicine at the University of Hawaii. He is an adjunct faculty member at the Tripler Army Medical Center and is compensated on a fee-for-service basis for teaching in the Psychiatry Residency Program. He receives compensation for his work as a psychiatry director of the American Board of Psychiatry and Neurology, Inc. He has no other relevant financial or fiduciary interests to report.

Michele C. Balas, Ph.D., R.N., C.C.R.N., is the Associate Dean of Research and Dorothy Hodges Olson Distinguished Professor of Nursing at the University of Nebraska Medical Center College of Nursing. She was a steering committee member of the Society of Critical Care Medicine's ICU Liberation Collaborative. She is currently Co-Chair of the Society of Critical Care Medicine's Pain, Agitation/Sedation, Delirium, Immobility, and Sleep (PADIS) guidelines and the American Association of Critical Care Nurse's Healthy Work Environment Collaborative. Her research is currently funded by the National Institutes of Health under award numbers 1 UG3 HL165740-01A1, 1 R01 NR020707-01, and 1 R01 HD103811-01. She has received past honoraria from Ceribell.

Robert Boland, M.D., receives compensation for his work as a psychiatry director of the American Board of Psychiatry and Neurology, Inc. He is a consultant for MCG Health, where he participates in peer review of care guidelines; however, Dr. Boland is not involved in guideline development. He has no other relevant financial or fiduciary interests.

Javier I. Escobar, M.D., M.Sc., is Emeritus Professor of Psychiatry at Rutgers University and Professor, Robert Stempel College of Public Health & Social Work, Florida International University (FIU). He receives a part-time salary from FIU as well as research funds from NIMH through the University of California at Los Angeles and the University of Texas at San Antonio. He reports no conflicts of interest with his work on this guideline.

Thomas Heinrich, M.D., is employed as a Professor of Psychiatry and Family Medicine by the Medical College of Wisconsin. In addition, he receives compensation for work as an Associate Medical Director at Network Health. He occasionally receives honoraria for Accreditation Council for Graduate Medical Education–compliant continuing medical education presentations. He reports no conflicts of interest with his work on this guideline.

Maga Jackson-Triche, M.D., M.S.H.S., is employed as the Department of Psychiatry Vice Chair for Adult Behavioral Health and as Vice President of Adult Behavioral Health Services, University of California San Francisco (UCSF) Health, at the UCSF School of Medicine and Medical Center. She reports no conflicts of interest with her work on this guideline.

James L. Levenson, M.D., is the Rhona Arenstein Professor of Psychiatry and Professor of Medicine and Surgery at Virginia Commonwealth University School of Medicine, where he is also Chair of the Division of Consultation-Liaison Psychiatry and Vice-Chair of the Department of Psychiatry. He receives royalties from the APA for *The American Psychiatric Association Publishing Textbook of Psychosomatic Medicine and Consultation-Liaison Psychiatry* and the *Clinical Manual of Psychopharmacology in the Medically Ill* and previously received royalties from UpToDate. He received compensation from Virginia Premier Medicaid Health Plan for service on the Credentials and Pharmacy and Therapeutics committees. He receives no compensation from any pharmaceutical company or any other commercial enterprise relevant to guideline development.

Melissa Mattison, M.D., is employed by Massachusetts General Physicians Organization as the Chief of Hospital Medicine and Associate Professor of Medicine at Harvard Medical School. She receives royalties from UpToDate and compensation as a reviewer for *Practical Reviews in Hospital Medicine* and as a consultant for Teladoc. She reports no conflicts of interest pertaining to her participation in developing this guideline.

Joseph McCullen Truett, D.O., was employed by George Washington University Health Sciences as a Consultation Liaison Psychiatry Fellow at Inova Fairfax Hospital and as an Attending Psychiatrist with Cityblock Health in Washington, D.C. He is currently employed as a Telemedicine Lead Psychiatrist for Lyra Health. He reports no conflicts of interest pertaining to his participation in developing this guideline.

Mark A. Oldham, M.D., is an Associate Professor of Psychiatry at the University of Rochester Medical Center, where he is the Medical Director of PRIME Medicine, the proactive arm of the psychiatric consultation-liaison service. He serves as President-Elect and board member of the American Delirium Society and Deputy Editor of the *Journal of the Academy of Consultation-Liaison Psychiatry*. He is supported by K23 AG072383 from the National Institute on Aging and 23IPA1047969 from the American Heart Association.

Andreea Seritan, M.D., is employed as a Professor of Clinical Psychiatry and Neurology at the UCSF School of Medicine and UCSF Weill Institute for Neurosciences. She receives grant support from the NIMH and the California Department of Public Health. She reports no conflict of interest with her work on this guideline.

Individuals and Organizations That Submitted Comments

Abrar AbuHamdia
Saeed Ahmed, M.D.
Giuseppe Bellelli, M.D.
James Alan Bourgeois, O.D., M.D.
William Breitbart, M.D., FAPA, FACLP
Hemlata Charitar, M.D., Ph.D., FAPA
John W. Devlin, Pharm.D.
Angela Eke-Usim, M.D.
Inga Giske, D.N.P., PMHNP-BC, NE-BC
Leslie Hartley Gise, M.D.
Paige Hector, L.M.S.W.
Rahul Lauhan, M.D.
Alasdair MacLullich, M.R.C.P., Ph.D.
Alessandro Morandi, M.D., M.P.H.
Karin J. Neufeld, M.D., M.P.H., FRCPC, DABPN
Brenda T. Pun, D.N.P., R.N., FCCM
Samuel Reinfeld, D.O.
John Shemo, M.D.
Paula Trzepacz, M.D.
Mark van den Boogaard, Ph.D., R.N.
Leiv Otto Watne, M.D., Ph.D.

American Academy of Physician Associates
American Association of Psychiatric Pharmacists
American Psychiatric Association Council on Consultation-Liaison Psychiatry
American Psychiatric Association Council on Research
American Society for Adolescent Psychiatry
Canadian Psychiatric Association
National Association of Social Workers
National Association of State Mental Health Program Directors
National Task Group on Intellectual Disabilities and Dementia Practices
Royal Australian and New Zealand College of Psychiatrists
The Association of Medicine and Psychiatry